Current Clinical Strategies

Medicine

AHRQ Guidelines

10th Edition

Paul D. Chan, MD
Executive Editor

Copyright © 2014 Current Clinical Strategies Publishing. All rights reserved.

This book, or any parts thereof, may not be reproduced or stored in an information retrieval network without the written permission of the publisher. The reader is advised to consult the package insert and other references before using any therapeutic agent. The publisher disclaims any liability, loss, injury, or damage incurred as a consequence, directly or indirectly, of the use and application of any of the contents of this text.

Current Clinical Strategies Publishing
PO Box 1753
Blue Jay, CA 92317
E-mail: info@ccspublishing.com

Printed in USA

ISBN 978-1-881528-34-0

Table of Contents

Medical Documentation

History and Physical Examination

Identifying Data: Patient's name; age, race, sex. List the patient's significant medical problems. Name of informant (patient, relative).

Chief Compliant: Reason given by patient for seeking medical care and the duration of the symptom. List the patient's medical problems.

History of Present Illness (HPI): Describe the course of the patient's illness, including when it began, character of the symptoms, location where the symptoms began; aggravating or alleviating factors; pertinent positives and negatives. Describe past illnesses or surgeries, and past diagnostic testing.

Past Medical History (PMH): Past diseases, surgeries, hospitalizations; medical problems; history of diabetes, hypertension, peptic ulcer disease, asthma, myocardial infarction, cancer. In children include birth history, prenatal history, immunizations, and type of feedings.

Medications:

Allergies: Penicillin, codeine?

Family History: Medical problems in family, including the patient's disorder. Asthma, coronary artery disease, heart failure, cancer, tuberculosis.

Social History: Alcohol, smoking, drug usage. Marital status, employment situation. Level of education.

Review of Systems (ROS):

General: Weight gain or loss, loss of appetite, fever, chills, fatigue, night sweats.

Skin: Rashes, skin discolorations.

Head: Headaches, dizziness, masses, seizures.

Eyes: Visual changes, eye pain.

Ears: Tinnitus, vertigo, hearing loss.

Nose: Nose bleeds, discharge, sinus diseases.

Mouth and Throat: Dental disease, hoarseness, throat pain.

Respiratory: Cough, shortness of breath, sputum (color).

Cardiovascular: Chest pain, orthopnea, paroxysmal nocturnal dyspnea; dyspnea on exertion, claudication, edema, valvular disease.

Gastrointestinal: Dysphagia, abdominal pain, nausea, vomiting, hematemesis, diarrhea, constipation, melena (black tarry stools), hematochezia (bright red blood per rectum).

Genitourinary: Dysuria, frequency, hesitancy, hematuria, discharge.

Gynecological: Gravida/para, abortions, last menstrual period (frequency, duration), age of menarche, menopause; dysmenorrhea, contraception, vaginal bleeding, breast masses.

Endocrine: Polyuria, polydipsia, skin or hair changes, heat intolerance.

Musculoskeletal: Joint pain or swelling, arthritis, myalgias.

Skin and Lymphatics: Easy bruising, lymphadenopathy.

Neuropsychiatric: Weakness, seizures, memory changes, depression.

Physical Examination

General appearance: Note whether the patient appears ill, well, or malnourished.

Vital Signs: Temperature, heart rate, respirations, blood pressure.

Skin: Rashes, scars, macules.

Lymph Nodes: Cervical, supraclavicular, axillary, inguinal nodes; size, tenderness.

Head: Bruising, masses. Check fontanels in pediatric patients.

Eyes: Pupils equal round and react to light and accommodation (PERRLA); extraocular movements intact (EOMI), visual fields. Funduscopy (papilledema, arteriovenous nicking, hemorrhages); icterus, ptosis.

Ears: Acuity, tympanic membranes (dull, shiny, intact, injected, bulging).

Mouth and Throat: Mucus membrane color and moisture; oral lesions, dentition, pharynx, tonsils.

Neck: Jugulovenous distention (JVD) at 45 degrees, thyromegaly, lymphadenopathy, masses, bruits, abdominojugular reflux.

Chest: Equal expansion, tactile fremitus, percussion, auscultation, rhonchi, crackles, breath sounds, egophony.

Heart: Point of maximal impulse (PMI), thrills (palpable turbulence); regular rate and rhythm (RRR), first and second heart sounds (S1, S2); gallops (S3, S4), murmurs (grade 1-6), pulses (graded 0-2+).

Breast: Dimpling, tenderness, masses, nipple discharge; axillary masses.

Abdomen: Contour (flat, scaphoid, obese, distended); scars, bowel sounds, bruits, tenderness, masses, liver span by percussion; hepatomegaly, splenomegaly; guarding, rebound, percussion note, costovertebral angle tenderness (CVAT).

Genitourinary: Inguinal masses, hernias, scrotum, testicles, varicoceles.

Pelvic Examination: Vaginal mucosa, cervical discharge, uterine size, masses, adnexal masses, ovaries.

Extremities: Joint swelling, range of motion, edema (grade 1-4+); cyanosis, clubbing, edema (CCE); pulses (radial, ulnar, femoral, popliteal, posterior tibial, dorsalis pedis).

Rectal Examination: Sphincter tone, masses, fissures; test for occult blood, prostate (nodules, tenderness, size).

Neurological: Mental status and affect; gait, strength (graded 0-5); touch sensation, pressure, pain, position and vibration; deep tendon reflexes (biceps, triceps, patellar, ankle; graded 0-4+); Romberg test (stand erect with arms outstretched and eyes closed).

Cranial Nerve Examination:

I: Smell

II: Vision and visual fields

III, IV, VI: Pupil responses to light, extraocular eye movements, ptosis

V: Facial sensation, ability to open jaw against resistance, corneal reflex.

VII: Close eyes tightly, smile, show teeth

VIII: Hears watch tic; Weber test (lateralization of sound with tuning fork on top of head); Rinne test (air conduction last longer than bone conduction with tuning fork on mastoid process)

IX, X: Palette moves in midline when patient says "ah."

XI: Shoulder shrug and turn head against resistance

XII: Stick out tongue in midline

Labs: Electrolytes (sodium, potassium, bicarbonate, chloride, BUN, creatinine), CBC (hemoglobin, hematocrit, WBC count, platelets, differential); X-rays, ECG, urine analysis (UA), liver function tests.

Assessment (Impression): Assign a number to each problem and discuss separately. Discuss differential diagnosis and give reasons that support the working diagnosis; give reasons for excluding other diagnoses.

Plan: Describe therapeutic plan for each numbered problem, including
  testing, laboratory studies, medications, and antibiotics.

Admission Check List

1. **Call and request** old chart, ECG, and X-rays.
2. **Stat labs:** CBC, Chem 7, troponin, INR, PTT, C&S, ABG, UA.
3. **Labs:** Toxicology screens and drug levels.
4. **Cultures:** Blood culture x 2, urine and sputum culture (before initiating
   antibiotics), sputum Gram stain, urinalysis.
5. **CXR, ECG**, diagnostic studies.
6. **Discuss case** with resident, attending, and family.

Progress Notes

Daily progress notes should summarize developments in a patient's
  hospital course, problems that remain active, plans to treat those
  problems, and arrangements for discharge.

Progress Note

Date/time:
Subjective: Any problems and symptoms of the patient should be
  charted. Appetite, pain, or insomnia may be included.
Objective:
  General appearance.
  Vitals, including highest temperature over past 24 hours. Fluid I/O
  (inputs and outputs), including oral, parenteral, urine, and stool
  volumes.
  Physical exam, including chest and abdomen, with attention to active
  problems.
Labs: Include new test results and circle abnormal values.
Current medications: List all medications and dosages.
Assessment and Plan: A separate assessment and plan should be
  written for each problem.

Procedure Note

A procedure note should be written in the chart when a procedure is performed.

Procedure Note
Date and time: **Procedure:** **Indications:** **Patient Consent:** Document that the indications and risks were explained to the patient and that the patient consented: "The patient understands the risks of the procedure and consents in writing." **Lab tests:** Relevant labs, such as the INR and CBC, chemistry. **Anesthesia:** Local with 2% lidocaine. **Description of Procedure:** Briefly describe the procedure, including sterile prep, anesthesia method, patient position, devices used, anatomic location of procedure, and outcome. **Complications and Estimated Blood Loss (EBL):** **Disposition:** Describe how the patient tolerated the procedure. **Specimens:** Describe any specimens obtained and labs tests which were ordered.

Discharge Note

The discharge note should be written in the patient's chart prior to discharge.

Discharge Note
Date/time: **Diagnoses:** **Treatment:** Briefly describe treatment provided during hospitalization, including surgical procedures and antibiotic therapy. **Studies Performed:** Electrocardiograms, CT scans. **Discharge Medications:** **Follow-up Arrangements:**

Discharge Summary

Patient's Name and Medical Record Number:
Date of Admission:
Date of Discharge:
Admitting Diagnosis:
Discharge Diagnosis:
Attending or Ward Team Responsible for Patient:
Surgical Procedures, Diagnostic Tests, Invasive Procedures:
Brief History, Pertinent Physical Examination, and Laboratory Data:
　　Describe the course of the patient's disease up to the time that the

patient came to the hospital, including physical exam and laboratory data.

Hospital Course: Describe the course of the patient's illness while in the hospital, including evaluation, treatment, medications, and outcome of treatment.

Discharged Condition: Describe improvement or deterioration in the patient's condition, and describe present status of the patient.

Disposition: Describe any the situation to which the patient will be discharged (home, nursing home), and indicate who will take care of patient.

Discharged Medications: List medications and instructions given to the patient.

Discharged Instructions and Follow-up Care: Date of return for follow-up care at clinic; diet, activity.

Problem List: List the patient's problems.

Copies: Send copies to attending, clinic, consultants.

Prescription Writing

- Patient's name:
- Date:
- Drug name, dosage form, dose, route, frequency (include concentration for oral liquids or mg strength for oral solids): Amoxicillin 125mg/5mL 5 mL PO tid
- Quantity to dispense:
- Refills: If appropriate
- Signature

12 Medical Documentation

Advanced Cardiovascular Life Support

Adult Basic Life Support

Unresponsive?
No breathing or no normal breathing or gasping only.

↓

Activate emergency response system → Get Defibrillator

↓

Start CPR - 30 Compressions, Airway, 2 Breaths

PUSH HARD AND PUSH FAST

Check rhythm/shock if Ventricular Tachycardia or Ventricular Fibrillation Repeat every 2 minutes

Basic Life Support Algorithm

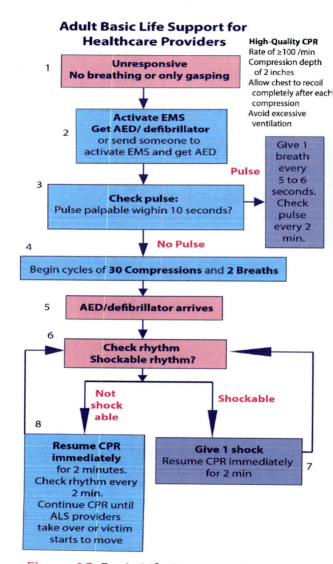

Figure 15. Basic Life Support Algorithm for Healthcare Providers

Adult Cardiac Arrest

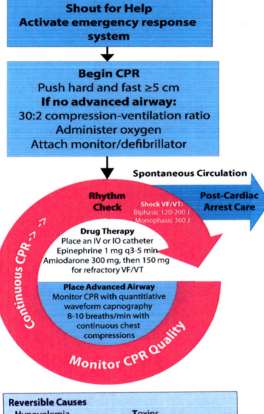

Shout for Help
Activate emergency response system

Begin CPR
Push hard and fast ≥5 cm
If no advanced airway:
30:2 compression-ventilation ratio
Administer oxygen
Attach monitor/defibrillator

Spontaneous Circulation

Rhythm Check

Shock VF/VT:
Biphasic 120-200 J
Monophasic 360 J

Post-Cardiac Arrest Care

Drug Therapy
Place an IV or IO catheter
Epinephrine 1 mg q3-5 min
Amiodarone 300 mg, then 150 mg
for refractory VF/VT

Place Advanced Airway
Monitor CPR with quantitiative
waveform capnography
8-10 breaths/min with
continuous chest
compressions

Continuous CPR

Monitor CPR Quality

Reversible Causes

Hypovolemia	**T**oxins
Hypoxia	**T**amponade, cardiac
Hydrogen ion (acidosis)	**T**ension pneumothorax
Hypo/hyperkalemia	**T**hrombosis coronary
Hypothermia	**T**hrombosis, pulmonary

Adult Cardiac Arrest Algorithm

Acute Coronary Syndromes

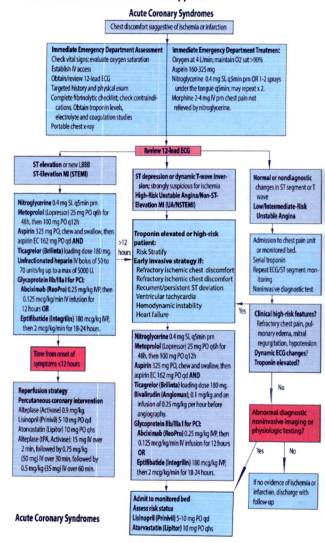

Chest discomfort suggestive of ischemia or infarction

Immediate Emergency Department Assessment
Check vital signs; evaluate oxygen saturation
Establish IV access
Obtain/review 12-lead ECG
Targeted history and physical exam
Complete fibrinolytic checklist; check contraindications. Obtain troponin levels,
electrolyte and coagulation studies
Portable chest x-ray

Immediate Emergency Department Treatment:
Oxygen at 4 L/min; maintain O2 sat >90%
Aspirin 160-325 mg
Nitroglycerine 0.4 mg SL q5min prn OR 1-2 sprays
under the tongue q5min; may repeat x 2.
Morphine 2-4 mg IV prn chest pain not
relieved by nitroglycerine.

Review 12-lead ECG

ST elevation or new LBBB
ST-Elevation MI (STEMI)

ST depression or dynamic T-wave inversion; strongly suspicious for ischemia
High-Risk Unstable Angina/Non-ST-Elevation MI (UA/NSTEMI)

Normal or nondiagnostic changes in ST segment or T wave
Low/Intermediate-Risk Unstable Angina

Nitroglycerine 0.4 mg SL q5min prn
Metoprolol (Lopressor) 25 mg PO q6h for
48h, then 100 mg PO q12h
Aspirin 325 mg PO, chew and swallow, then
aspirin EC 162 mg PO qd **AND**
Ticagrelor (Brilinta) loading dose 180 mg.
Unfractionated heparin IV bolus of 50 to
70 units/kg up to a max of 5000 U.
Glycoprotein IIb/IIIa I for PCI:
Abciximab (ReoPro) 0.25 mg/kg IVP, then
0.125 mcg/kg/min IV infusion for
12 hours **OR**
Eptifibatide (Integrilin) 180 mcg/kg IVP,
then 2 mcg/kg/min for 18-24 hours.

Troponin elevated or high-risk patient:
Risk Stratify
Early invasive strategy if:
Refractory ischemic chest discomfort
Refractory ischemic chest discomfort
Recurrent/persistent ST deviation
Ventricular tachycardia
Hemodynamic instability
Heart failure

>12 hours

Admission to chest pain unit
or monitored bed.
Serial troponin
Repeat ECG/ST segment monitoring
Noninvasive diagnostic test

Clinical high-risk features?
Refractory chest pain, pulmonary edema, mitral
regurgitation, hypotension
Dynamic ECG changes?
Troponin elevated?

Yes

Time from onset of symptoms ≤12 hours

Nitroglycerine 0.4 mg SL q5min prn
Metoprolol (Lopressor) 25 mg PO q6h for
48h, then 100 mg PO q12h
Aspirin 325 mg PO, chew and swallow, then
aspirin EC 162 mg PO qd **AND**
Ticagrelor (Brilinta) loading dose 180 mg.
Bivalirudin (Angiomax), 0.1 mg/kg and an
infusion of 0.25 mg/kg per hour before
angiography.
Glycoprotein IIb/IIIa I for PCI:
Abciximab (ReoPro) 0.25 mg/kg IVP, then
0.125 mcg/kg/min IV infusion for 12 hours
OR
Eptifibatide (Integrilin) 180 mcg/kg IVP,
then 2 mcg/kg/min for 18-24 hours.

No

Reperfusion strategy
Percutaneous coronary intervention
Alteplase (Activase) 0.9 mg/kg.
Lisinostatin (Lipitor) 10 mg PO qd
Atorvastatin (Lipitor) 10 mg PO qhs
Alteplase (tPA, Activase): 15 mg IV over
2 min, followed by 0.75 mg/kg
(50 mg) IV over 30 min, followed by
0.5 mg/kg (35 mg) IV over 60 min.

Abnormal diagnostic noninvasive imaging or physiologic testing?

Yes

No

If no evidence of ischemia or infarction, discharge with follow-up

Admit to monitored bed
Assess risk status
Lisinopril (Prinivil) 5-10 mg PO qd
Atorvastatin (Lipitor) 10 mg PO qhs

Acute Coronary Syndromes

Adult Cardiac Arrest with No Pulse

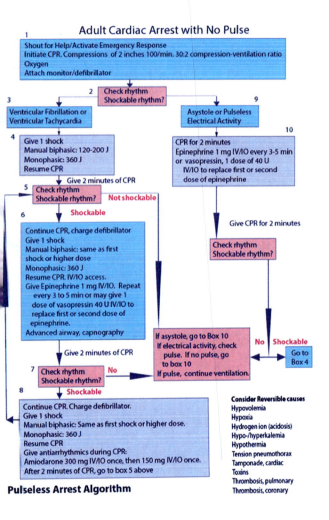

1
Shout for Help/Activate Emergency Response
Initiate CPR. Compressions of 2 inches 100/min. 30:2 compression-ventilation ratio
Oxygen
Attach monitor/defibrillator

2 Check rhythm
Shockable rhythm?

3
Ventricular Fibrillation or
Ventricular Tachycardia

9
Asystole or Pulseless
Electrical Activity

4
Give 1 shock
Manual biphasic: 120-200 J
Monophasic: 360 J
Resume CPR

10
CPR for 2 minutes
Epinephrine 1 mg IV/IO every 3-5 min
or vasopressin, 1 dose of 40 U
IV/IO to replace first or second
dose of epinephrine

Give 2 minutes of CPR

5 Check rhythm
Shockable rhythm?   **Not shockable**

Shockable

6
Continue CPR, charge defibrillator
Give 1 shock
Manual biphasic: same as first
shock or higher dose
Monophasic: 360 J
Resume CPR. IV/IO access.
Give Epinephrine 1 mg IV/IO. Repeat
every 3 to 5 min or may give 1
dose of vasopressin 40 U IV/IO to
replace first or second dose of
epinephrine.
Advanced airway, capnography

Give CPR for 2 minutes

Check rhythm
Shockable rhythm?

If asystole, go to Box 10
If electrical activity, check
pulse. If no pulse, go
to box 10
If pulse, continue ventilation.

No   Shockable
Go to
Box 4

Give 2 minutes of CPR

7 Check rhythm
Shockable rhythm?   **No**

Shockable

8
Continue CPR. Charge defibrillator.
Give 1 shock
Manual biphasic: Same as first shock or higher dose.
Monophasic: 360 J
Resume CPR
Give antiarrhythmics during CPR:
Amiodarone 300 mg IV/IO once, then 150 mg IV/IO once.
After 2 minutes of CPR, go to box 5 above

Consider Reversible causes
Hypovolemia
Hypoxia
Hydrogen ion (acidosis)
Hypo-/hyperkalemia
Hypothermia
Tension pneumothorax
Tamponade, cardiac
Toxins
Thrombosis, pulmonary
Thrombosis, coronary

Pulseless Arrest Algorithm

Bradycardia with Pulses

Bradycardia: Heart rate <50 beats/min and inadequate heart rate for clinical condition

Maintain patent Airway, assist Breathing as needed Give oxygen Monitor ECG, pulse oximeter and blood pressure	Secure IV access Review history **Search for underlying cause:** Hypoxemia, hypovolemia, hyperkalemia, hypokalemia?

Signs or symptoms of Poor Perfusion caused by bradycardia? (eg, confusion, delirium, lethargy, chest pain, hypotension or other signs of shock)

Adequate Perfusion

Poor Perfusion

Observe and Monitor

Reminders
- If pulseless arrest develops, go to Pulseless Arrest Algorithm
- Search for and treat possible contributing factors:
  Hypovolemia
  Hypoxia
  Hydrogen ion (acidosis)
  Hypo/hyperkalemia
  Hypothermia
  Toxins
  Tamponade, cardiac
  Tension pneumothorax
  Thrombosis (coronary or pulmonary)
  Trauma (hypovolemia, increased ICP)

- Atropine 0.5 mg IV, repeat q3-5min to a total dose of 3 mg.
- Initiate transcutanous pacing for high-degree block (type II second or 3rd degree heart block, wide complex escape beats, MI/ischemia, denervated heart (transplant), new bundle branch block)
- Consider dopamine 2-10 mcg/kg per min IV infusion or epinephrine 2-10 mcg/min IV infusion while awaiting pacer or if pacing ineffective

Initiate transvenous pacing
Treat contributing causes
Obtain cardiology consultation

Bradycardia Algorithm (with patient not in cardiac arrest).

Tachycardia >150 bpm with Palpable Pulses

Assess Airway, Breathing, Circulation
Administer 100% oxygen by mask or nasal canula
Attach electrocardiographic monitor and identify rhythm. Monitor pulse oximeter, blood pressure.
Identify and treat rthe cause of the tachycardia (hypovolemia, hypoxia, toxins, tamponade, thrombosis)
Review history and examine patient

Determine if the patient is stable
Unstable includes hypotension, heart failure, chest pain, decreased mental status.

Unstable →

SYNCHRONIZED CARDIOVERSION
Initiate IV access and give midazolam (Versed) 2-5 mg IVP if conscious
Narrow regular 50-100 J
Narrow irregular: 120-200 J
Wide regular: 100 J
Wide irregular: Unsynchronized 1 20-200 J
If regular narrow complex, give adenosine 12 mg rapid IV push followed by NS flush.
If pulseless arrests develops, go to the Pulseless Arrest Algorithm.

Stable

Establish IV access
Obtain 12-lead ECG
Is QRS narrow (<0.12 sec)?

Narrow QRS (<0.12 sec)   Wide QRS (≥0.12 sec)

IV access and check 12-lead ECG.
Perform vagal maneuvers: Carotid massage, Valsalva maneuver.
If regular, administer **Adenosine** 6 mg rapid IV push, followed by NS flush.
If no conversion, repeat 12 mg.
Control rate with Diltiazem, 15 mg IV over 2 min; then 5-15 mg/hr IV or esmolol 500 mcg/kg; 50-300 mcg/kg/min.

IV access. Check 12-lead ECG.
Adenosine: If regular and monomorphic, give 6 mg, rapid IV push (may repeat 12 mg once).
Procainamide 20-50 mg/min until suppression of arrhythmia, hypotension develops, QRS duration increases >50%, or max 17 mg/kg given. Maintenance infusion of 1-4 mg/min. Contraindicated if prolonged QT or heart failure.
Amiodarone 150 mg IV over 10 min. Repeat as needed for recurrent VT. Follow by maintenance infusion of 1 mg/min for 6 hours.
Sotalol 100 mg IV (1.5 mg/kg) over 5 minutes. Avoid if prolonged QT interval.

Treat contributing factors:
Hypovolemia
Hypoxia
Hydrogen ion (acidosis)
Hypo/hyperkalemia
Hypoglycemia
Hypothermia
Tamponade, cardiac
Toxins
Tension pneumothorax
Thrombosis (coronary artery or pulmonary)
Trauma (hypovolemia, increased ICP)

Suspected Ischemic Stroke

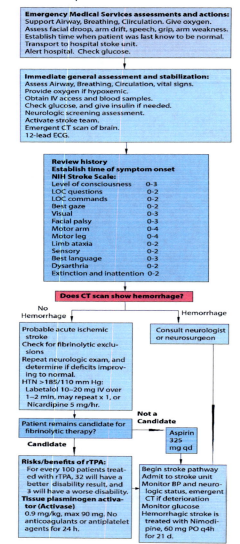

Emergency Medical Services assessments and actions:
Support Airway, Breathing, Cilrculation. Give oxygen.
Assess facial droop, arm drift, speech, grip, arm weakness.
Establish time when patient was last know to be normal.
Transport to hospital stoke unit.
Alert hospital. Check glucose.

Immediate general assessment and stabilization:
Assess Airway, Breathing, Circulation, vital signs.
Provide oxygen if hypoxemic.
Obtain IV access and blood samples.
Check glucose, and give insulin if needed.
Neurologic screening assessment.
Activate stroke team.
Emergent CT scan of brain.
12-lead ECG.

Review history
Establish time of symptom onset
NIH Stroke Scale:

Level of consciousness	0-3
LOC questions	0-2
LOC commands	0-2
Best gaze	0-2
Visual	0-3
Facial palsy	0-3
Motor arm	0-4
Motor leg	0-4
Limb ataxia	0-2
Sensory	0-2
Best language	0-3
Dysarthria	0-2
Extinction and inattention	0-2

Does CT scan show hemorrhage?

No Hemorrhage → | Hemorrhage →

Probable acute ischemic stroke
Check for fibrinolytic exclusions
Repeat neurologic exam, and determine if deficits improving to normal.
HTN >185/110 mm Hg:
  Labetalol 10–20 mg IV over 1–2 min, may repeat x 1, or Nicardipine 5 mg/hr.

Consult neurologist or neurosurgeon

Patient remains candidate for fibrinolytic therapy?

Not a Candidate →

Aspirin 325 mg qd

Candidate

Risks/benefits of rTPA:
For every 100 patients treated with rTPA, 32 will have a better disability result, and 3 will have a worse disability.
Tissue plasminogen activator (Activase)
0.9 mg/kg, max 90 mg. No anticoagulants or antiplatelet agents for 24 h.

Begin stroke pathway
Admit to stroke unit
Monitor BP and neurologic status, emergent CT if deterioration
Monitor glucose
Hemorrhagic stroke is treated with Nimodipine, 60 mg PO q4h for 21 d.

Acute Ischemic Stroke Algorithm

Cardiovascular Disorders

ST-Segment Elevation Myocardial Infarction

1. **Admit to:** Coronary care unit
2. **Diagnosis:** ST-segment elevation myocardial infarction
3. **Condition:**
4. **Vital Signs:** q1h. Call physician if pulse >90 mmHg,<60 mmHg; BP >150/90, <90/60; R>25/min, <12; T >38.5°C.
5. **Activity:** Bed rest with bedside commode.
7. **Nursing:** If patient has chest pain, obtain 12-lead ECG and call physician.
8. **Diet:** Cardiac diet, 1-2 gm sodium, low-fat, low-cholesterol diet.
9. **IV Fluids:** D5W at TKO
10. **Special Medications:**
    -Oxygen 2-4 L/min by NC.
    -Aspirin 325 mg PO, chew and swallow immediately, then aspirin EC 162 mg PO qd **AND**
    -Ticagrelor (Brilinta) 180 mg loading dose; Maintenance: 90 mg twice daily **AND**
    -Nitroglycerin SL, 0.4 mg (0.15-0.6 mg) SL q5min until pain free (up to 3 tabs) **OR** Nitroglycerin spray (0.4 mg/aerosol spray) 1-2 sprays under the tongue q 5min; may repeat x 2.

Glycoprotein IIb/IIIa Blockers for Planned PCI:
    -Abciximab (ReoPro) 0.25 mg/kg IVP, then 0.125 mcg/kg/min IV infusion for 12 hours **OR**
    -Eptifibatide (Integrilin) 180 mcg/kg IVP, then 2 mcg/kg/min for 18-24 hours.

Anticoagulant for Planned PCI:
    -Unfractionated heparin IV bolus of 50 to 70 units/kg up to a maximum of 5000 units.

Thrombolytic Therapy (within first 6 hours of onset of chest pain)
Absolute Contraindications to Thrombolytics: Active internal bleeding, aortic dissection, intracranial neoplasm, previous intracranial hemorrhagic stroke at any time, other strokes or cerebrovascular events within 1 year, head trauma, pregnancy, non-compressible vascular puncture, hypertension (>180/110 mm Hg).

A. **Alteplase (tPA, tissue plasminogen activator, Activase):**
    1. 15 mg IV push over 2 min, followed by 0.75 mg/kg (50 mg) IV infusion over 30 min, followed by 0.5 mg/kg (35 mg) IV infusion over 60 min (total dose 100 mg).
    2. **Labs:** INR/PTT, CBC, fibrinogen.

Beta-Blockers: Contraindicated in cardiogenic shock.
    -Metoprolol (Lopressor) 25 mg PO q6h for 48h, then 100 mg PO q12h; hold if heart rate <60/min or systolic BP <100 mm Hg **OR**
    -Atenolol (Tenormin), 50-100 mg PO qd.

Angiotensin Converting Enzyme Inhibitor (within the first 24 hours of onset of chest pain):
    -Lisinopril (Zestril, Prinivil) 2.5-5 mg PO qd; titrate to 10-20 mg qd.

Long-Acting Nitrates:
    -Nitroglycerin patch 0.2 mg/hr qd. Allow for nitrate-free period to prevent tachyphylaxis.

-Isosorbide dinitrate (Isordil) 10-60 mg PO tid [5,10,20, 30,40 mg] **OR**
-Isosorbide mononitrate (Imdur) 30-60 mg PO qd.
Aldosterone Receptor Blockers:
-Eplerenone (Inspra) 24 mg PO qd
-Spironolactone (Aldactone) 25 mg PO qd
Statins:
-Atorvastatin (Lipitor) 10 mg PO qhs **OR**
-Rosuvastatin (Crestor) 10 mg PO qhs.
11. **Symptomatic Medications:**
-Morphine sulfate 2-4 mg IV push prn chest pain.
-Acetaminophen (Tylenol) 325-650 mg PO q4-6h prn headache.
-Lorazepam (Ativan) 1-2 mg PO tid-qid prn anxiety
-Zolpidem (Ambien) 5-10 mg qhs prn insomnia.
-Docusate (Colace) 100 mg PO bid.
-Ondansetron (Zofran) 2-4 mg IV q4h prn nausea or vomiting.
-Famotidine (Pepcid) 20 mg IV/PO bid **OR**
-Lansoprazole (Prevacid) 30 mg qd.
12. **Extras:** ECG stat and in 12h and in AM, portable CXR, impedance cardiography, echocardiogram, exercise stress test, cardiovascular magnetic resonance imaging.. Cardiology consult.
13. **Labs:** SMA7 and 12, magnesium. Troponin, CBC, INR/PTT, UA.

Non-ST Segment Elevation Myocardial Infarction (NSTEMI) and Unstable Angina

1. **Admit to:** Coronary care unit
2. **Diagnosis:** Acute coronary syndrome
3 **Condition:**
4. **Vital Signs:** q1h. Call physician if pulse 90 mmHg,<60 mmHg; BP >150/90, <90/60; R>25/min, <12; T >38.5°C.
5. **Activity:** Bed rest with bedside commode.
7. **Nursing:** Guaiac stools. If patient has chest pain, obtain 12-lead ECG and call physician.
8. **Diet:** Cardiac diet, 1-2 gm sodium, low fat, low cholesterol.
9. **IV Fluids:** D5W at TKO
10. **Special Medications:**
-Oxygen 2-4 L/min by NC.
-Aspirin 325 mg PO, chew and swallow, then aspirin EC 162 mg PO qd **AND**
-Ticagrelor (Brilinta) 180 mg loading dose; Maintenance: 90 mg twice daily
-Nitroglycerin SL, 0.4 mg SL q5min until pain-free (up to 3 tabs) **OR**
-Nitroglycerin spray (0.4 mg/aerosol spray) 1-2 sprays under the tongue q 5min; may repeat 2 times.
Anticoagulant for Planned PCI:
-Bivalirudin (Angiomax), IV bolus of 0.1 mg/kg and an infusion of 0.25 mg/kg per hour before angiography.
Glycoprotein IIb/IIIa Blockers for Planned PCI:
-Abciximab (ReoPro) 0.25 mg/kg IVP, then 0.125 mcg/kg/min IV infusion for 12 hours **OR**
-Eptifibatide (Integrilin) 180 mcg/kg IVP, then 2 mcg/kg/min for 18-24 hours.

Beta-Blockers: Contraindicated in cardiogenic shock.
-Metoprolol (Lopressor) 25 mg PO q6h for 48h, then 100 mg PO q12h; keep HR <60/min, hold if systolic BP <100 mm Hg **OR**
-Atenolol (Tenormin) 50-100 mg PO qd **OR**
-Esmolol (Brevibloc) 500 mcg/kg IV over 1 min, then 50 mcg/kg/min IV infusion, titrated to heart rate >60 bpm (max 300 mcg/kg/min).
Angiotensin Converting Enzyme Inhibitors:
-Lisinopril (Zestril, Prinivil) 2.5-5 mg PO qd; titrate to 10-20 mg qd **OR**
-Benazepril (Lotensin) 10 mg qd **OR**
-Rampril (Altace) 5-10 mg qd **OR**
-Perindopril (Aceon) 4-8 mg qd.
Long-Acting Nitrates:
-Nitroglycerin patch 0.2 mg/hr qd. Allow for nitrate-free period to prevent tachyphylaxis.
-Isosorbide dinitrate (Isordil) 10-60 mg PO tid [5,10,20, 30,40 mg] **OR**
-Isosorbide mononitrate (Imdur) 30-60 mg PO qd.
Statins:
-Atorvastatin (Lipitor) 10 mg PO qhs **OR**
-Rosuvastatin (Crestor) 10 mg PO qd **OR**
-Pravastatin (Pravachol) 40 mg PO qhs **OR**
-Simvastatin (Zocor) 40 mg PO qhs **OR**
-Lovastatin (Mevacor) 20 mg PO qhs **OR**
-Fluvastatin (Lescol)10-20 mg PO qhs.
11. **Symptomatic Medications:**
-Morphine sulfate 2-4 mg IV push prn chest pain.
-Acetaminophen (Tylenol) 325-650 mg PO q4-6h prn headache.
-Lorazepam (Ativan) 1-2 mg PO tid-qid prn anxiety.
-Zolpidem (Ambien) 5-10 mg qhs prn insomnia.
-Docusate (Colace) 100 mg PO bid.
-Ondansetron (Zofran) 2-4 mg IV q4h prn N/V.
-Famotidine (Pepcid) 20 mg IV/PO bid **OR**
-Lansoprazole (Prevacid) 30 mg qd.
12. **Extras:** ECG stat and in 12h and in AM, portable CXR, impedance cardiography, echocardiogram, exercise stress test, cardiovascular magnetic resonance imaging. Cardiology consult.
13. **Labs:** SMA7 and 12, magnesium. Troponin, CBC, INR/PTT, UA.

Heart Failure Due to Systolic Dysfunction

1. **Admit to:**
2. **Diagnosis:** Heart failure due to systolic dysfunction
3. **Condition:**
4. **Vital Signs:** q1h. Call physician if P >120; BP >150/100 <80/60; T >38.5°C; R >25/min, <10.
5. **Activity:** Bed rest with bedside commode.
6. **Nursing:** Daily weights, measure inputs and outputs. Head-of-bed at 45 degrees.
7. **Diet:** 1-2 gm salt, cardiac diet.
8. **IV Fluids:** Saline lock with flush q shift.
9. **Special Medications:**
-Oxygen 2-4 L/min by NC.

Diuretics:
- Furosemide (Lasix) 10-160 mg IV qd-bid or 20-80 mg PO qAM-bid [20, 40, 80 mg] or 10-40 mg/hr IV infusion **OR**
- Torsemide (Demadex) 10-40 mg IV or PO qd; max 200 mg/day [5, 10, 20, 100 mg] **OR**
- Bumetanide (Bumex) 0.5-1 mg IV q2-3h until response; then 0.5-1.0 mg IV q8-24h (max 10 mg/d); or 0.5-2.0 mg PO qAM.

ACE Inhibitors:
- Lisinopril (Zestril, Prinivil) 5-40 mg PO qd [5, 10, 20, 40 mg] **OR**
- Quinapril (Accupril) 5-10 mg PO qd x 1 dose, then 20-80 mg PO qd in 1 to 2 divided doses [5, 10, 20, 40 mg] **OR**
- Benazepril (Lotensin) 10-20 mg PO qd-bid, max 80 mg/d [5, 10, 20, 40 mg] **OR**
- Fosinopril (Monopril) 10-40 mg PO qd, max 80 mg/d [10, 20 mg] **OR**
- Ramipril (Altace) 2.5-10 mg PO qd, max 20 mg/d [1.25, 2.5, 5, 10 mg].
- Captopril (Capoten) 6.25-50 mg PO q8h [12.5, 25,50,100 mg] **OR**
- Enalapril (Vasotec) 1.25-5 mg slow IV push q6h or 2.5-20 mg PO bid [5,10,20 mg] **OR**
- Moexipril (Univasc) 7.5 mg PO qd x 1 dose, then 7.5-15 mg PO qd-bid [7.5, 15 mg tabs] **OR**
- Trandolapril (Mavik) 1 mg qd x 1 dose, then 2-4 mg qd [1, 2, 4 mg tabs].

Angiotensin-II Receptor Blockers:
- Candesartan (Atacand) 8-16 mg qd-bid [4, 8, 16, 32 mg].
- Losartan (Cozaar) 25-50 mg bid [25, 50 mg].
- Irbesartan (Avapro) 150 mg qd, max 300 mg qd [75, 150, 300 mg].
- Valsartan (Diovan) 80 mg qd; max 320 mg qd [80, 160 mg].
- Telmisartan (Micardis) 40-80 mg qd [40, 80 mg].

Adosterone Receptor Blockers:
- Spironolactose (Aldactone) 25 mg PO qd.
- Eplerenone (Inspra) 25 mg PO qd.

Beta-Blockers:
- Carvedilol (Coreg) 3.125 mg PO bid, then slowly increase every 2 weeks to target dose of 25-50 mg bid [tab 3.125, 6.25, 12.5, 25 mg] **OR**
- Metoprolol (Lopressor) start at 12.5 mg bid, then slowly increase to target dose of 100 mg bid [50, 100 mg]. Metoprolol XL (Toprol XL) 50-100 mg PO qd. **OR**
- Bisoprolol (Zebeta) start at 1.25 mg qd, then slowly increase to target of 5-10 mg qd [5,10 mg].

Digoxin (Lanoxin) 0.125-0.25 mg PO or IV qd [0.125, 0.25, 0.5 mg].

Inotropic Agents:
- Dobutamine (Dobutrex) 2.5-10 mcg/kg/min IV, max of 14 mcg/kg/min (500 mg in 250 mL D5W, 2 mcg/mL) **OR**
- Dopamine (Intropin) 3-15 mcg/kg/min IV (400 mg in 250 cc D5W, 1600 mcg/mL), titrate to CO >4, CI >2; systolic >90 mmHg **OR**
- Milrinone (Primacor) 0.375 mcg/kg/min IV infusion (40 mg in 200 mL NS, 0.2 mg/mL); titrate to 0.75 mcg/kg/min; arrhythmogenic; may cause hypotension.

Vasodilators:
- Isosorbide dinitrate/hydralazine (BiDil), 20 mg/37.5 mg tabs, 1-2 tabs tid; decreases mortality in black patients with heart failure when added to standard treatment.

Potassium:
-KCL (Micro-K) 20-60 mEq PO qd if the patient is taking loop diuretics.

Pacing:
-Synchronized biventricular pacing if ejection fraction <40% and QRS duration >135 msec.

10. Symptomatic Medications:
-Morphine sulfate 2-4 mg IV push prn dyspnea or anxiety.
-Heparin 5000 U SQ q12h or enoxaparin (Lovenox) 1 mg/kg SC q12h.
-Docusate (Colace) 100-200 mg PO qhs.
-Famotidine (Pepcid) 20 mg IV/PO q12h **OR**
-Lansoprazole (Prevacid) 30 mg qd.

11. Extras: CXR PA and LAT, ECG now and repeat if chest pain or palpitations; echocardiogram, exercise stress test. Cardiovascular magnetic resonance imaging.

12. Labs: Basic metabolic panel, basic chemistry, CBC; B-type natriuretic peptide (BNP), troponin, TSH, free T4, ferritin and TIBC. Repeat Basic metabolic panel in AM. UA.

Atrial Fibrillation

1. Admit to:

2. Diagnosis: Atrial fibrillation

3. Condition:

4. Vital Signs: q1h. Call physician if BP >160/90 mmHg, <90/60 mmHg; apical pulse >130/min, <50; R >25/min, <10; T >38.5°C

5. Activity: Bedrest with bedside commode.

6. Nursing: Pulse oximeter.

7. Diet: Low fat, low cholesterol, no caffeine.

8. IV Fluids: D5W at TKO.

9. Special Medications:

Anticoagulation:
-Dabigatran (Pradaxa) 150 mg twice daily for at least one month after cardioversion.
-Warfarin (Coumadin) 5 mg PO once a day for two days. Check the INR on the third day. Modify subsequent doses to achieve a target INR of 2.5 (2.0 to 3.0).
-Heparin (unfractionated) 80 U/kg IVP, then 18 U/kg/hr IV infusion. Check PTT 6 hours after initial bolus; adjust q6h until PTT 1.5-2.0 times control (50-80 sec).

Cardioversion (if unstable):
1. Midazolam (Versed) 2-5 mg IV push.
2. If stable, cardiovert with synchronized synchronized cardioversion at 120 to 200 joules for biphasic devices and 200 joules for monophasic devices.

Initial Rate Control with Mild to Moderate Symptoms:
-Metoprolol (Lopressor) is given as an intravenous bolus of 2.5 to 5.0 mg over two minutes. The dose may be repeated at five minute intervals up to a total of 15 mg as needed. Then 50-100 mg PO bid, or metoprolol XL (Toprol-XL) 50-100 mg PO qd **OR**
-Esmolol (Brevibloc) bolus of 0.5 mg/kg is infused over one minute, followed by 50 µg/kg per min. If, after four minutes, the response is inadequate, another bolus is given followed by an infusion of 100 µg/kg per min. If, after four minutes, the response is still inadequate,

a third and final bolus can be given followed by an infusion of 150 µg/kg per min. If necessary, the infusion can be increased to a maximum of 200 µg/kg per min after another four minutes **OR**

-Atenolol (Tenormin) 25 mg of atenolol per day and gradually increase the daily dose to 100 mg, and sometimes 200 mg, if necessary.

Calcium channel blockers

-Diltiazem (Cardizem) bolus of 0.25 mg/kg (20 mg) IV over two minutes; in 15 minutes, if first dose does not produce heart rate <100 beats/min, a second bolus of 0.35 mg/kg (25 mg) is given over 2 min; continuous infusion of 5 to 15 mg/h. Oral diltiazem 30 mg PO qid, max 360 to 480 mg daily (ie, 90 to 120 mg qid). Sustained release diltiazem is given qd or divided into two doses.

-Verapamil (Calan) 40 mg three or four times per day increased to a maximum of 360 mg/day in divided doses. Sustained release verapamil is given once per day.

-Digoxin (Lanoxin) loading dose: 0.25 mg IV every 2 hours, up to 1.5 mg within 24 hours. For non-acute situations, administer 0.5 mg PO qd for 2 days followed by maintenance IV, oral: 0.125-0.375 mg once daily.

-Procainamide (Pronestyl) Loading dose: Infuse 20-50 mg/minute or 100 mg every 5 minutes until arrhythmia controlled, hypotension occurs, QRS complex widens by 50%, or 17 mg/kg is given. Follow with 1-4 mg/min IV.

10. **Symptomatic Medications:**
    -Lorazepam (Ativan) 1-2 mg PO tid prn anxiety.
11. **Extras:** Portable CXR, ECG; repeat if chest pain; transthoracic echocardiogram Cardiology consult.
12. **Labs:** CBC, Basic metabolic panel, chemistry panel & 12, serial troponin levels, Mg, TSH, Free T4. UA.

Ventricular Arrhythmias

1. **Ventricular Fibrillation and Tachycardia:**
   -**If unstable (see ACLS protocol):** Defibrillate with unsynchronized 200 J, then 300 J.
   -Oxygen 100% by mask.
   -Amiodarone (Cordarone) 300 mg in 100 mL of D5W, IV infusion over 10 min, then 900 mg in 500 mL of D5W, at 1 mg/min for 6 hrs, then at 0.5 mg/min thereafter; or 400 mg PO q8h x 14 days, then 200-400 mg qd.
   -**Also see "other antiarrhythmics" below.**
2. **Torsades de Pointes Ventricular Tachycardia:**
   -Correct underlying causes, including hypomagnesemia, hypokalemia, quinidine, procainamide, disopyramide, moricizine, amiodarone, sotalol, ibutilide, phenothiazine, haloperidol, tricyclic and tetracyclic antidepressants, ketoconazole, itraconazole, bepridil.
   -Magnesium sulfate 1-4 gm in 100 mL IV bolus over 5-15 min, or infuse 3-20 mg/min for 7-48h until QTc interval <440 msec.
   -Consider ventricular pacing and/or cardioversion.

. Other Antiarrhythmics:

Class I:
- Moricizine (Ethmozine) 200-300 mg PO q8h, max 900 mg/d [200, 250, 300 mg].

Class Ia:
- Quinidine gluconate (Quinaglute) 324-648 mg PO q8-12h [324 mg].
- Procainamide (Procan, Procanbid)
  IV: 15 mg/kg IV loading dose at 20 mg/min, followed by 2-4 mg/min continuous IV infusion.
  PO: 500 mg (nonsustained release) PO q2h x 2 doses, then Procanbid 1-2 gm PO q12h [500, 1000 mg].
- Disopyramide (Norpace, Norpace CR) 100-300 mg PO q6-8h [100, 150, mg] or disopyramide CR 100-150 mg PO bid [100, 150 mg].

Class Ib:
- Mexiletine (Mexitil) 100-200 mg PO q8h, max 1200 mg/d [150, 200, 250 mg].
- Tocainide (Tonocard) loading 400-600 mg PO, then 400-600 mg PO q8-12h (1200-1800 mg/d) PO in divided doses q8-12h [400, 600 mg].
- Phenytoin (Dilantin), loading dose 100-300 mg IV given as 50 mg in NS over 10 min IV q5min, then 100 mg IV q5min prn.

Class Ic:
- Flecainide (Tambocor) 50-100 mg PO q12h, max 400 mg/d [50, 100, 150 mg].
- Propafenone (Rythmol) 150-300 mg PO q8h, max 1200 mg/d [150, 225, 300 mg].

Class II:
- Propranolol (Inderal) 1-3 mg IV in NS (max 0.15 mg/kg) or 20-80 mg PO tid-qid [10, 20, 40, 60, 80 mg]; propranolol-LA (Inderal-LA), 80-120 mg PO qd [60, 80, 120, 160 mg]
- Esmolol (Brevibloc) loading dose 500 mcg/kg over 1 min, then 50-200 mcg/kg/min IV infusion
- Atenolol (Tenormin) 50-100 mg/d PO [25, 50, 100 mg].
- Nadolol (Corgard) 40-100 mg PO qd-bid [20, 40, 80, 120, 160 mg].
- Metoprolol (Lopressor) 50-100 mg PO bid-tid [50, 100 mg], or metoprolol XL (Toprol-XL) 50-200 mg PO qd [50, 100, 200 mg].

Class III:
- Amiodarone (Cordarone), PO loading 400-1200 mg/d in divided doses for 2-4 weeks, then 200-400 mg PO qd (5-10 mg/kg) [200 mg] or amiodarone (Cordarone) 300 mg in 100 mL of D5W, IV infusion over 10-20 min, then 900 mg in 500 mL of D5W, at 1 mg/min for 6 hrs, then at 0.5 mg/min thereafter.
- Sotalol (Betapace) 40-80 mg PO bid, max 320 mg/d in 2-3 divided doses [80, 160 mg].

4. **Extras:** CXR, ECG, Holter monitor, signal averaged ECG, cardiology consult.
5. **Labs**: Basic metabolic panel, basic chemistry, Mg, calcium, CBC, TSH, free T4, drug levels. UA.

Hypertensive Emergencies

1. **Admit to:**
2. **Diagnosis:** Hypertensive emergencies
3. **Condition:**
4. **Vital Signs:** q30min until BP controlled, then q4h.
5. **Activity:** Bed rest
6. **Nursing:** Intra-arterial BP monitoring, daily weights, inputs and outputs.
7. **Diet:** Clear liquids.
8. **IV Fluids:** D5W at TKO.
9. **Special Medications:**
   -Nitroprusside (Nipride) 0.25 to 0.5 mcg/kg per minute. Maximum 8 to 10 mcg/kg per minute; higher doses should generally be avoided or limited to a maximum duration of 10 minutes.
   -Nitroglycerin 5 mcg/min, maximum of 100 mcg/min.
   -Clevidipine (Cleviprex) 1 mg/hour, which can be increased as necessary to a maximum of 21 mg/hour.
   -Labetalol (Trandate, Normodyne) 20 mg IV bolus (0.25 mg/kg), then 20-80 mg boluses IV q10-15min, titrate to desired BP or continuous IV infusion of 1.0-2.0 mg/min, titrate to desired BP.
   -Fenoldopam (Corlopam) 0.1 mcg/kg/min IV infusion. Adjust dose by 0.025-0.05 mcg/kg/min q15min to max 0.3 mcg/kg/min. [10 mg in 250 mL D5W].
   -Nicardipine (Cardene IV) 5 mg/hr IV infusion, increase rate by 2.5 mg/hr every 15 min up to 15 mg/hr (25 mg in D5W 250 mL).
   -Enalaprilat (Vasotec IV) 1.25- 5.0 mg IV q6h. Do not use in presence of acute myocardial infarction or bilateral renal stenosis.
   -Esmolol (Brevibloc) 500 mcg/kg/min IV infusion for 1 minute, then 50 mcg/kg/min; titrate by 50 mcg/kg/min increments to 300 mcg/kg/min (2.5 gm in D5W 250 mL).
   -Phentolamine (pheochromocytoma), 5-10 mg IV, repeated as needed up to 20 mg.
   -Trimethaphan (Arfonad [dissecting aneurysm]) 2-4 mg/min IV infusion (500 mg in 500 mL of D5W).
   -Nifedipine XL (Procardia XL) 30 mg PO once daily **OR**
   -Metoprolol XL (Toprol XL) 50 mg daily **OR**
   -Ramipril (Altace) 10 mg once daily.
10. **Symptomatic Medications:**
    -Acetaminophen (Tylenol) 325-650 mg PO q4-6h prn headache.
    -Zolpidem (Ambien) 5-10 mg qhs prn insomnia.
    -Docusate sodium (Colace) 100-200 mg PO qhs.
11. **Extras:** Portable CXR, ECG, echocardiogram.
12. **Labs:** CBC, basic metabolic panel, troponin, UA with micro. TSH, free T4, 24h urine for metanephrine. Plasma catecholamines, urine drug screen.

Hypertension

I. Initial Diagnostic Evaluation of Hypertension
- **A. 15-Lead electrocardiography** may document evidence of ischemic heart disease, rhythm and conduction disturbances, or left ventricular hypertrophy.
- **B. Screening labs.** Complete blood count, glucose, potassium, calcium, creatinine, BUN, uric acid, and fasting lipid panel.
- **C. Urinalysis.** Glucose, protein.
- **D.** Urine albumin-to-creatinine, echocardiography. Duplex Doppler renal ultrasonography, plasma fractionated metanephrines.

II. Antihypertensive Drugs JNC-8 Guidelines
- **A. ≥60 years old:** Pharmacologic treatment should be initiated at a systolic SBP of 150 mmHg or a diastolic BP of 90 mmHg.
- **B. < 60 years old:** Initiate pharmacologic treatment at a DBP of 90 mmHg or an SBP of 140 mmHg and treat to goals.
- **C. Diabetes or CKD:** Initiate pharmacologic treatment at an SBP of 140 mmHg or a DBP of 90 mmHg.
- **D. Nonblacks:** Initial treatment is thiazide-type diuretic, calcium channel blocker, ACE inhibitor or angiotensin receptor blocker.
- **E. Blacks:** Initial treatment is thiazide-type diuretic or a CCB.
- **F. Chronic Kidney Disease:** Initial treatment is ACE inhibitor or an ARB.
- **G. Thiazide Diuretics**
  1. **Hydrochlorothiazide (HCTZ, HydroDiuril)**, 12.5-25 mg qd [25 mg].
  2. **Chlorothiazide (Diuril)** 250 mg qd [250, 500 mg].
  3. **Thiazide/Potassium Sparing Diuretic Combinations**
     a. Maxzide (hydrochlorothiazide 50/triamterene 75 mg) 1 tab qd.
     b. Moduretic (hydrochlorothiazide 50 mg/amiloride 5 mg) 1 tab qd.
     c. Dyazide (hydrochlorothiazide 25 mg/triamterene 37.5) 1 cap qd.
- **H. Beta-Adrenergic Blockers**
  1. **Cardioselective Beta-Blockers**
     a. **Atenolol (Tenormin)** initial dose 50 mg qd, then 50-100 mg qd, max 200 mg/d [25, 50, 100 mg].
     b. **Metoprolol XL (Toprol XL)** 100-200 mg qd [50, 100, 200 mg tab ER].
     c. **Bisoprolol (Zebeta)** 2.5-10 mg qd; max 20 mg qd [5,10 mg].
  2. **Non-Cardioselective Beta-Blocker**
     a. **Propranolol LA (Inderal LA)**, 80-160 mg qd [60, 80, 120, 160 mg].
- **I. Angiotensin-Converting Enzyme (ACE) Inhibitors**
  1. **Ramipril (Altace)** 2.5-10 mg qd, max 20 mg/day [1.25, 2.5, 5, 10 mg].
  2. **Lisinopril (Zestril, Prinivil)** 10-40 mg qd [2.5, 5, 10, 20, 40 mg].
  3. **Quinapril (Accupril)** 20-80 mg qd [5, 10, 20, 40 mg].
  4. **Benazepril (Lotensin)** 10-40 mg qd, max 80 mg/day [5, 10, 20, 40 mg].
  5. **Fosinopril (Monopril)** 10-40 mg qd [10, 20 mg].
  6. **Enalapril (Vasotec)** 5-40 mg qd, max 40 mg/day [2.5, 5, 10, 20 mg].
  7. **Moexipril (Univasc)** 7.5-15 mg qd [7.5 mg].
- **J. Angiotensin Receptor Blockers**

1. **Losartan (Cozaar)** 25-50 mg bid [25, 50 mg].
2. **Valsartan (Diovan)** 80-160 mg qd; max 320 mg qd [80, 160 mg].
3. **Irbesartan (Avapro)** 150 mg qd; max 300 mg qd [75, 150, 300 mg].
4. **Candesartan (Atacand)** 8-16 mg qd-bid [4, 8, 16, 32 mg].
5. **Telmisartan (Micardis)** 40-80 mg qd [40, 80 mg].

K. **Calcium Channel Blockers**
1. **Diltiazem SR (Cardizem SR)** 60-120 mg bid [60, 90, 120 mg] or **Cardizem CD** 180-360 mg qd [120, 180, 240, 300 mg].
2. **Nifedipine XL (Procardia-XL, Adalat-CC)** 30-90 mg qd [30, 60, 90 mg].
3. **Verapamil SR (Calan SR, Covera-HS)** 120-240 mg qd [120, 180, 240 mg].
4. **Amlodipine (Norvasc)** 2.5-10 mg qd [2.5, 5, 10 mg].
5. **Felodipine (Plendil)** 5-10 mg qd [2.5, 5, 10 mg].

Syncope

1. **Admit to:** Monitored bed
2. **Diagnosis:** Syncope
3. **Condition:**
4. **Vital Signs:** q1h. Call physician if BP >160/90, <90/60; P >120, <50; R>25/min, <10
5. **Activity:** Bed rest.
6. **Nursing:**
7. **Diet:** Regular
8. **IV Fluids:** Normal saline at TKO.
9. **Special medications:**
High-Grade AV Block with Syncope:
-Atropine 1 mg IV x 2.
-Isoproterenol 0.5-1 mcg/min initially, then slowly titrate to 10 mcg/min IV infusion (1 mg in 250 mL NS).
-Transthoracic pacing.
Drug-Induced Syncope:
-Discontinue vasodilators, centrally acting hypotensive agents, phenothiazines, antidepressants, and alcohol use.
Vasovagal Syncope:
-Scopolamine 1.5 mg transdermal patch q3 days.
Postural Syncope:
-Midodrine (ProAmatine) 2.5 mg PO tid, then increase to 5-10 mg PO tid [2.5, 5 mg]; contraindicated in coronary artery disease.
-Fludrocortisone 0.1-1.0 mg PO qd.
10. **Symptomatic Medications:**
-Acetaminophen (Tylenol) 325-650 mg PO q4-6h prn headache.
-Docusate sodium (Colace) 100-200 mg PO qhs.
11. **Extras:** CXR, ECG, 24h Holter monitor, electrophysiologic study, tilt test, CT/MRI, EEG, echocardiogram.
12. **Labs:** CBC, Basic metabolic panel, basic chemistry, troponin, Mg, calcium, drug levels. UA, urine drug screen.

Pulmonary Disorders

Asthma

1. **Admit to:**
2. **Diagnosis:** Exacerbation of asthma
3. **Condition:**
4. **Vital Signs:** q6h. Call physician if P >140; R >30, <10; T >38.5°C; pulse oximeter <90%
5. **Activity:** Up as tolerated.
6. **Nursing:** Pulse oximeter, bedside peak flow rate before and after bronchodilator treatments.
7. **Diet:** Regular, no caffeine.
8. **IV Fluids:** D5 ½ NS at 125 cc/h.
9. **Special Medications:**
   -Oxygen 2 L/min by NC. Keep O_2 sat >94%.

Beta-Agonists, Acute Treatment:
   -Albuterol (Ventolin) 2.5 to 5 mg by continuous flow nebulization every 20 minutes for three doses, then 2.5 to 10 mg every one to four hours as needed. Or continuous nebulization, 10 to 15 mg over one hour. **OR**
   -Albuterol (Ventolin) MDI with a spacer, 4 puffs every 10 minutes or 8 puffs every 20 minutes for up to four hours, then 4 to 8 puffs every one to four hours as needed.

Systemic Corticosteroids:
   -Methylprednisolone (Solu-Medrol) 60 to 80 mg every 6 to 12 hours for patients in the intensive care unit to 40 to 60 mg every 12 to 24 hours for patients not requiring intensive care **OR**
   -Prednisone 20-60 mg PO qAM.

Ipratropium (Atrovent) nebulization 500 mcg q20 min for 3 doses, then as needed. Or MDI 8 inhalations every 20 minutes, then as needed. May be helpful to patients with severe exacerbations in the emergency department.

Magnesium sulfate, 2 grams in 100 mL normal saline over 20 minutes, is suggested for patients who have life-threatening exacerbations.

Helium-oxygen (heliox) gas mixtures for acute, severe exacerbations may be helpful but is not standard therapy.

Maintenance Inhaled Corticosteroids:
   -Advair Diskus (fluticasone/salmeterol) one puff bid [doses of 100/50 mcg, 250/50 mcg, and 500/50 mcg]. Not appropriate for acute attacks.
   -Beclomethasone (Beclovent) MDI 4-8 puffs bid, with spacer 5 min after bronchodilator, followed by gargling with water.
   -Triamcinolone (Azmacort) MDI 2 puffs tid-qid or 4 puffs bid.
   -Flunisolide (AeroBid) MDI 2-4 puffs bid.
   -Fluticasone (Flovent) 2-4 puffs bid (44 or 110 mcg/puff).

Maintenance Treatment:
   -Salmeterol (Serevent) 2 puffs bid; not effective for acute asthma because of delayed onset of action.
   -Pirbuterol (Maxair) MDI 2 puffs q4-6h prn.
   -Bitolterol (Tornalate) MDI 2-3 puffs q1-3min, then 2-3 puffs q4-8h prn.
   -Fenoterol (Berotec) MDI 3 puffs, then 2 bid-qid.

10. Symptomatic Medications:
  -Docusate sodium (Colace) 100 mg PO qhs.
  -Famotidine (Pepcid) 20 mg IV/PO q12h **OR**
  -Lansoprazole (Prevacid) 30 mg qd.
  -Acetaminophen (Tylenol) 325-650 mg PO q4-6h prn headache.
11. Extras: Portable CXR, ECG, pulmonary function tests before and after bronchodilators.
12. Labs: ABG, CBC with eosinophil count, SMA7, B-type natriuretic peptide (BNP). Theophylline level stat and after 24h of infusion. Sputum Gram stain, C&S.

Chronic Obstructive Pulmonary Disease

1. Admit to:
2. Diagnosis: Acute exacerbation of COPD
3. Condition:
4. Vital Signs: q4h. Call physician if P >130; R >30, <10; T >38.5°C; O_2 saturation <90%.
5. Activity: Up as tolerated; bedside commode.
6. Nursing: Pulse oximeter. Measure peak flow with portable peak flow meter bid. No sedatives.
7. Diet: No added salt diet. Push fluids.
8. IV Fluids: D5 ½ NS with 20 mEq KCL/L at 125 cc/h.
9. Special Medications:
  -Oxygen 24-35% by Venturi mask, keep O_2 saturation 90-94%.
Beta-Agonists, Acute Treatment:
  -Albuterol (Ventolin) 2.5 mg (diluted to a total of 3 mL) by nebulizer every one to four hours as needed or MDI 4-8 puffs q4-6h.
  -Ipratropium (Atrovent) 500 mcg by nebulizer every four hours as needed. Or two puffs by MDI with a spacer every four hours as needed.
Glucocorticoids and Anticholinergics:
  -Methylprednisolone (Solu-Medrol) 60-125 mg IV q6h. **Followed by:**
  -Prednisone 30-60 mg PO qd.
  -Ipratropium (Atrovent) MDI 2 puffs tid-qid.
  -Triamcinolone (Azmacort) MDI 2 puffs qid or 4 puffs bid.
  -Beclomethasone (Beclovent) MDI 4-8 puffs bid with spacer, followed by gargling with water **OR**
  -Flunisolide (AeroBid) MDI 2-4 puffs bid **OR**
  -Fluticasone (Flovent) 2-4 puffs bid (44 or 110 mcg/puff).
Acute Bronchitis
  -Levofloxacin (Levaquin) 500 mg PO/IV qd [250, 500 mg] **OR**
  -Cefepime (Maxipime) 1-2 gm IV q12h **OR**
  -Ceftazidime (Fortaz) 1 gm IV q8h **OR**
  -Piperacillin-tazobactam (Zosyn) 3.375 gm IV/PB q6h **OR**
  -Trimethoprim/sulfamethoxazole (Septra DS) 160/800 mg PO bid or 160/800 mg IV q12h (10-15 mL in 100 cc D5W tid) **OR**
  -Azithromycin (Zithromax) 500 mg x 1, then 250 mg PO qd x 4 or 500 mg IV q24h **OR**
  -Clarithromycin (Biaxin) 250-500 mg PO bid.
10. Symptomatic Medications:
  -Docusate sodium (Colace) 100 mg PO qhs.

-Famotidine (Pepcid) 20 mg IV/PO bid **OR**
-Lansoprazole (Prevacid) 30 mg qd.
-Acetaminophen (Tylenol) 325-650 mg PO q4-6h prn headache.
11. Extras: Portable CXR, PFTs with bronchodilators, ECG.
12. Labs: ABG, CBC, SMA7, UA. Theophylline level stat and after 12-24h of infusion. Sputum Gram stain and C&S, alpha 1 antitrypsin level.

Hemoptysis

1. **Admit to:** Intensive care unit
2. **Diagnosis:** Hemoptysis
3. **Condition:**
4. **Vital Signs:** q1-6h. Orthostatic BP and pulse. Call physician if BP >160/90, <90/60; P >130, <50; R>25/min, <10; T >38.5°C; O₂ sat <90%.
5. **Activity:** Bed rest with bedside commode. Keep patient in lateral decubitus, Trendelenburg's position, bleeding side down.
6. **Nursing:** Measure all sputum and expectorated blood, suction prn. O₂ at 100% by mask, pulse oximeter. Discontinue sedatives. Foley to closed drainage.
7. **Diet:** NPO
8. **IV Fluids:** 1 L of NS wide open (≥6 gauge), then transfuse PRBC. Then infuse D5 ½ NS at 125 cc/h.
9. **Special Medications:**
   -Transfuse 2-4 U PRBC wide open.
   -Trimethoprim/sulfamethoxazole (Septra DS) 160/800 mg PO bid or 160/800 mg IV q12h (10-15 mL in 100 cc D5W tid) **OR**
   -Cefuroxime (Zinacef) 750 mg IV q8h **OR**
   -Ampicillin/sulbactam (Unasyn) 1.5 gm IV q6h
10. **Extras:** CXR PA, LAT, ECG, contrast CT, bronchoscopy. PPD, pulmonary and thoracic surgery consults.
11. **Labs:** Type and cross 2-4 U PRBC. ABG, CBC, platelets, SMA7 and 12. Anti-glomerular basement antibody, rheumatoid factor, complement, anti-nuclear cytoplasmic antibody. Sputum Gram stain, C&S, AFB culture, and cytology. UA, INR/PTT, von Willebrand Factor. Repeat CBC q8h.

Anaphylaxis

1. **Admit to:**
2. **Diagnosis:** Anaphylaxis
3. **Condition:**
4. **Vital Signs:** q1-4h; call physician if BP systolic >160, <90; diastolic >90 mmHg, <60 mmHg; P >120, <50; R>25/min, <10; T >38.5°C
5. **Activity:** Bedrest
6. **Nursing:** O₂ at 6 L/min by NC or mask. Keep patient in Trendelenburg's position, No. 4 or 5 endotracheal tube at bedside. Foley to closed drainage.
7. **Diet:** NPO
8. **IV Fluids:** 2 IV lines. Normal saline 1 L over 10 minutes, then D5 ½ NS at 125 cc/h.

9. Special Medications:
Bronchodilators:
-Epinephrine (1:1000) 0.3-0.5 mL IM q10min or 1-4 mcg/min IV. Epinephrine, 0.3 mL of 1:1000 solution, may be injected SQ at site of allergen injection **OR**
-Albuterol (Ventolin) 0.5%, 0.5 mL in 2.5 mL NS q30min by nebulizer prn
Corticosteroids:
-Methylprednisolone (Solu-Medrol) 250 mg IV x 1, then 125 mg IV q6h **OR**
-Hydrocortisone 200 mg IV x 1, then 100 mg q6h, followed by oral prednisone 60 mg PO qd, tapered over 5 days.
Antihistamines:
-Diphenhydramine (Benadryl) 25-50 mg PO/IV q4-6h **OR**
-Cetirizine (Zyrtec) 5-10 mg PO qd.
-Cimetidine (Tagamet) 300 mg PO/IV q6-8h.
Pressors:
-Norepinephrine (Levophed) 8-12 mcg/min IV, titrate to systolic 100 mm Hg (8 mg in 500 mL D5W) **OR**
-Dopamine (Intropin) 5-20 mcg/kg/min IV.
10. Extras: Portable CXR, ECG, allergy consult.
11. Labs: CBC, Basic metabolic panel, basic chemistry.

Pleural Effusion

1. Admit to:
2. Diagnosis: Pleural effusion
3. Condition:
4. Vital Signs: q shift. Call physician if BP >160/90, <90/60; P>120, <50; R>25/min, <10; T >38.5°C
5. Activity:
6. Diet: Regular.
7. IV Fluids: D5W at TKO
8. Extras: CXR PA and LAT, repeat after thoracentesis; left and right lateral decubitus x-rays, ECG, ultrasound, PPD; pulmonary consult.
9. Labs: CBC, Basic metabolic panel, basic chemistry, protein, albumin, amylase, INR/PTT, UA, cryptococcal antigen.
Thoracentesis:
Tube 1: LDH, protein, amylase, triglyceride, glucose (10 mL).
Tube 2: Gram stain, C&S, AFB, fungal C&S (20-60 mL, heparinized).
Tube 3: Cell count and differential (5-10 mL, EDTA).
Syringe: pH (2 mL collected anaerobically, heparinized on ice).
Bag or Bottle: Cytology.

Hematologic Disorders

Anticoagulant Overdose

Unfractionated Heparin Overdose:
1. Discontinue heparin infusion.
2. Protamine sulfate, 1 mg IV for every 100 units of heparin infused in preceding hour, dilute in 25 mL fluid, and give IV over 10 min (max 50 mg in 10 min period).

Low-Molecular-Weight Heparin (Enoxaparin) Overdose:
-Protamine sulfate 1 mg IV for each 1 mg of enoxaparin given. Repeat protamine 0.5 mg IV for each 1 mg of enoxaparin. If bleeding continues
after 2-4 hours. Measure factor Xa.

Warfarin (Coumadin) Overdose:
- Discontinue coumadin.

Partial Reversal:
-Vitamin K (Phytonadione), 0.5-1.0 mg IV/SQ. Check INR in 24 hours, and repeat vitamin K dose if INR remains elevated.

Minor Bleeds:
-Vitamin K (Phytonadione), 5-10 mg IV/SQ q12h, titrated to desired INR.

Serious Bleeds:
-Vitamin K (Phytonadione), 10-20 mg in 50-100 mL fluid IV over 30-60 min (check INR q6h until corrected) **AND**
-Fresh frozen plasma 2-4 units x 1.
-Type and cross match for 2 units of PRBC, and transfuse wide open.
-Cryoprecipitate 10 U x 1 if fibrinogen is less than 100 mg/dL.

Labs: CBC, platelets, PTT, INR.

Deep Vein Thrombosis

1. **Admit to:**
2. **Diagnosis:** Deep vein thrombosis
3. **Condition:**
4. **Vital Signs:** q shift. Call physician if BP systolic >160, <90 diastolic, >90 mmHg, <60 mmHg; P >120, <50; R>25/min, <10; T >38.5°C.
5. **Activity:** Bed rest with legs elevated.
6. **Nursing:** Guaiac stools, warm packs to leg prn; measure calf circumference qd; no intramuscular injections.
7. **Diet:** Regular
8. **IV Fluids:** D5W at TKO
9. **Special Medications:**

Anticoagulation:
-Dalteparin (Fragmin) 200 units/kg SubQ once daily **OR**
-Enoxaparin (Lovenox) inpatient treatment 1 mg/kg/dose SubQ every 12 hours or 1.5 mg/kg once daily. Outpatient treatment: 1 mg/kg/dose every 12 hours. Start warfarin on the first or second treatment day and continue enoxaparin until INR is ≥ for at least 24 hours (usually 5-7 days) **OR**
-Heparin (unfractionated) 80 U/kg IVP, then 18 U/kg/hr IV infusion. Check

PTT 6 hours after initial bolus; adjust q6h until PTT 1.5-2.0 times control (50-80 sec). Dose should be sufficient to prolong the aPTT to a range that corresponds to a plasma heparin level of 0.3 to 0.7 units/mL by an anti-Xa assay.

- Treatment with LMW heparin , heparin, or fondaparinux should be continued for at least five days, and oral anticoagulation with a vitamin K antagonist should be initiated simultaneously, and both agents should be overlapped for at least 5days. The heparin or fondaparinux can be discontinued on day 5 or 6 if the INR has been in the therapeutic range for at least 24 hours or two consecutive days.
- Fondaparinux (Arixtra) <50 kg: 5 mg SQ once daily; 50-100 kg: 7.5 mg SC once daily; >100 kg: 10 mg SQ once daily.
- Warfarin (Coumadin) 5-10 mg PO qd x 2-3 d; maintain INR 2.5 (range: 2.0 to 3.0). Coumadin is initiated on the first or second day [tab 1, 2, 2.5, 3 4, 5, 6, 7.5, 10 mg].
- Tissue plasminogen activator (tPA) 100 mg IV over two hours. Anticoagulant therapy should be discontinued during thrombolytic infusion. When the thrombolytic is complete, an aPTT should be measured. Heparin should be resumed without a loading dose when the aPTT is less than twice its upper limit of normal.

10. **Symptomatic Medications:**
    - Propoxyphene/acetaminophen (Darvocet N100) 1-2 tab PO q3-4h prn pain **OR**
    - Hydrocodone/acetaminophen (Vicodin), 1-2 tab q4-6h PO prn pain.
    - Docusate sodium (Colace) 100 mg PO qhs.
    - Famotidine (Pepcid) 20 mg IV/PO q12h **OR**
    - Lansoprazole (Prevacid) 30 mg qd.
    - Zolpidem (Ambien) 5-10 mg qhs prn insomnia.
11. **Extras:** CXR PA and LAT, ECG; compression ultrasonography of legs. Chest CT scan.
12. **Labs:** d-dimer, CBC, INR/PTT, basic metabolic panel. Antiphospholipid antibodies. UA with dipstick for blood. PTT 6h after bolus and q4-6h until PTT is 1.5-2.0 x control then qd. INR at initiation of warfarin and qd.

Pulmonary Embolism

1. **Admit to:**
2. **Diagnosis:** Pulmonary embolism
3. **Condition:**
4. **Vital Signs:** q1-4h. Call physician if BP >160/90, <90/60; P >120, <50; R >30, <10; T >38.5°C; O_2 sat < 90%
5. **Activity:** Bedrest with bedside commode
6. **Nursing:** Pulse oximeter, guaiac stools, O_2 at 2 L by NC. Antiembolism stockings. No intramuscular injections. Foley to closed drainage.
7. **Diet:** Regular
8. **IV Fluids:** Normal saline 1 L IV over 20 minutes, then 120 ml/h.

9. Special Medications:

Anticoagulation:

-Norepinephrine (Levophed) 2-8 mcg/min IV infusion (8 mg in 250 mL D5W). If hypotension does not resolve with intravenous fluids.

-Enoxaparin (Lovenox) 1 mg/kg of subcutaneously every 12 hours. Or 1.5 mg/kg subcutaneously once daily.

-Dalteparin (Fragmin) 200 international units/kg subcutaneously once daily (maximum 18,000 international units) for 30 days. Then 150 international units/kg once daily (maximum 18,000 international units).

-Fondaparinux (Arixtra) patients <50 kg: 5 mg SQ qd; patients 50 to 100 kg: 7.5 mg SQ qd; and patients >100 kg: 10 mg SQ qd.

-Warfarin (Coumadin) 5 mg PO qd for two days, then check INR on day 3 and adjust subsequent doses to achieve an INR of 2.5 (range 2.0 to 3.0). Warfarin can be initiated at the same time or after LMWH, UFH, or fondaparinux. Warfarin should be overlapped with LMWH, UFH, or fondaparinux for a minimum of five days and until the INR has been within the therapeutic range for at least 24 hours.

-Heparin IV bolus 5000-10,000 Units (100 U/kg) IVP, then 1000-1500 U/h IV infusion (20 U/kg/h) [25,000 U in 500 mL D5W (50 U/mL)]. Check PTT 6 hours after initial bolus; adjust q6h until PTT 1.5-2 times control (60-80 sec). Overlap heparin and Coumadin for at least 4 days and discontinue heparin when INR has been 2.0-3.0 for two consecutive days OR SQ unfractionated heparin 5000 units IV bolus, followed by SQ doses of 250 units/kg twice daily.

-Warfarin (Coumadin) 5-10 mg PO qd for 2-3 d, then 2-5 mg PO qd. Maintain INR of 2.0-3.0. [tab 1, 2, 2.5, 3, 4, 5, 6, 7.5, 10 mg].

Thrombolytics for hemodynamic compromise:

-Alteplase (recombinant tissue plasminogen activator, Activase): 100 mg IV infusion over 2 hours. Discontinue anticoagulant until tPA finished. Then start heparin at 15 U/kg/h to maintain PTT 1.5-2 x control.

10. Symptomatic Medications:

-Fentanyl 0.35 to 1.50 mcg/kg IV every 0.5 to 1 hour, and continuous intravenous infusion doses of 0.7 to 10 mcg/kg/hr.

-Docusate sodium (Colace) 100 mg PO qhs.

-Famotidine (Pepcid) 20 mg IV/PO q12h **OR**

-Lansoprazole (Prevacid) 30 mg qd.

11. Extras: CXR PA and LAT, ECG, chest CT scan; Doppler ultrasonography of lower extremities.

12. Labs: d-dimer CBC, INR/PTT, SMA7, ABG,. Antiphospholipid antibody. UA . PTT 6 hours after bolus and q4-6h.

Sickle Cell Acute Pain Episode

1. Admit to:

2. Diagnosis: Sickle cell acute pain episode

3. Condition:

4. Vital Signs: q shift.

5. Activity: Bedrest with bathroom privileges.

6. Nursing:

7. Diet: Regular diet, push oral fluids.

8. IV Fluids: D5 ½ NS at 100-125 mL/h.

9. Special Medications:

-Oxygen 2 L/min by NC or 30-100% by mask.

38 Sickle Cell Acute Pain Episode

-Morphine sulfate 5-10 mg IV/IM q2-4h prn pain **OR**
-Acetaminophen/codeine (Tylenol 3) 1-2 tabs PO q4-6h prn.
-Folic acid 1 mg PO qd.
-Penicillin V (prophylaxis), 250 mg PO qid [tabs 125,250,500 mg].
-Ondansetron (Zofran) 4 mg PO/IV q4-6h prn nausea or vomiting.

10. Symptomatic Medications:
-Zolpidem (Ambien) 5-10 mg qhs prn insomnia.
-Docusate sodium (Colace) 100-200 mg PO qhs.

Vaccination:
-Pneumovax before discharge 0.5 mL IM x 1 dose.
-Influenza vaccine (Fluogen) 0.5 mL IM once a year in the Fall.

11. Extras: CXR.

12. Labs: CBC, basic metabolic panel, blood C&S, reticulocyte count, blood type and screen, parvovirus titers. UA.

Infectious Diseases

Meningitis

1. **Admit to:**
2. **Diagnosis:** Meningitis.
3. **Condition:**
4. **Vital Signs:** q1h. Call physician if BP systolic >160/90 mmHg, <90/60; P >120/min, <50; R>25/min, <10; T >39°C or less than 36°C
   Activity: Bed rest with bedside commode.
5. **Nursing:** Respiratory isolation, lumbar puncture tray at bedside.
6. **Diet:** NPO
7. **IV Fluids:** D5 ½ NS at 125 cc/h with KCL 20 mEq/L.
8. **Special Medications:**
Empiric Therapy 15-50 years old:
   -Vancomycin 1 gm IV q12h **AND**
   -Ceftriaxone (Rocephin) 2 gm IV q12h (max 4 gm/d) **OR**
   Cefotaxime (Claforan) 2 gm IV q4h.
Empiric Therapy >50 years old, Alcoholic, Corticosteroids or Hematologic Malignancy or other Debilitating Condition:
   -Ampicillin 2 gm IV q4h **AND**
   -Cefotaxime (Claforan) 2 gm IV q6h **OR**
   Ceftriaxone (Rocephin) 2 gm IV q12h.
   -Use Vancomycin 1 gm IV q12h in place of ampicillin if drug-resistant pneumococcus is suspected.
10. **Symptomatic Medications:**
   -Dexamethasone (Decadron) 0.4 mg/kg IV q12h x 2 days with first dose of antibiotic.
   -Heparin 5000 U SC q12h or pneumatic compression stockings.
   -Famotidine (Pepcid) 20 mg IV/PO q12h.
   -Acetaminophen (Tylenol) 650 mg PO/PR q4-6h prn temp >39°C.
   -Docusate sodium 100-200 mg PO qhs.
11. **Extras:** CXR, ECG, CT scan.
12. **Labs:** CBC, Basic metabolic panel, basic chemistry. Blood C&S x 2. UA with micro, urine C&S. Antibiotic levels peak and trough after 3rd dose, VDRL.
Lumbar Puncture:
   CSF Tube 1: Gram stain, C&S for bacteria (1-4 mL).
   CSF Tube 2: Glucose, protein (1-2 mL).
   CSF Tube 3: Cell count and differential (1-2 mL).
   CSF Tube 4: Antigen tests for S. pneumoniae, H. influenzae (type B), N. -meningitides, E. coli, group B strep, VDRL, cryptococcal antigen, toxoplasma titers (8-10 mL).

Native Valve Endocarditis

1. **Admit to:**
2. **Diagnosis:** Infective endocarditis
3. **Condition:**
4. **Vital Signs:** q8h. Call physician if BP systolic >160/90, <90/60; P >120, <50; R>25/min, <10; T >38.5°C

5. **Activity:** Up ad lib, bathroom privileges.
6. **Diet:** Regular
7. **IV Fluids:** Saline lock with flush q shift.
8. **Special Medications:**

Empiric therapy no known immunodeficiency:
-Vancomycin (30 mg/kg per 24 h IV in two divided doses) for four to six weeks.

Viridans Streptococci and Streptococcus Bovis
-Penicillin G at a dose of 12 to 18 million units daily (continuously or in four to six equally divided doses) for four weeks **OR**
- Gentamicin 3 mg/kg per day or in two to three equally divided doses adjusted to give a peak serum level of 3 to 4 mcg/mL. plus (aqueous crystalline penicillin G or ceftriaxone) for two weeks.
-**Patients with mild penicillin allergy** can be treated with ceftriaxone. Patients with immediate-type penicillin hypersensitivity may be treated with vancomycin (30 mg/kg/d in two divided doses) for four weeks.

Pneumococcus:
-Penicillin G (24 million units per day either continuously or in four to six equally divided doses).

Enterococci:
-Gentamicin 3 mg/kg per 24 hours IV or IM in three equally divided doses for four to six weeks. **Plus one of the following:**
-Aqueous penicillin G 18 to 30 million units per 24 hours IV either continuously or in six equally divided doses for four to six weeks **OR**
-Ampicillin 12 g IV q24 hours in 6l divided doses for four to six weeks **OR**
-Vancomycin 30 mg/kg/24 hours IV in two equally divided doses for 4- 6 weeks; not to exceed 2 g per 24 hours.

Staphylococcal Endocarditis:
-Nafcillin 12 g IV daily in 4-6 divided doses **OR**
-Flucloxacillin (Floxapen) 2 g every four to six hours.
Penicillin allergy: Cefazolin (Ancef) 2 g intravenously every eight hours if there is no immediate-type allergy. Vancomycin, 15-20 mg/kg/dose every 8-12 hours for 6 weeks, is an alternative with immediate-type penicillin allergy.
Methicillin resistant: Vancomycin 15-20 mg/kg/dose every 8-12 hours for 6 weeks for six weeks.

HACEK Organisms:
-Ceftriaxone (Rocephin) 2 gm IV q24h, ampicillin-sulbactam , or ciprofloxacin for four weeks.

Other Gram-negative Organisms (E. Coli, Pseudomonas, or Mucoid Strains of Klebsiella or Serratia):
-Ceftriaxone (Rocephin) 2 g once daily IV **OR**
-Ciprofloxacin (Cipro) 400 mg q 12 IV.

Culture-negative Endocarditis
-Ampicillin-sulbactam plus gentamicin **OR**
-Vancomycin plus gentamicin plus ciprofloxacin for four to six weeks.
-Ceftriaxone (Rocephin) 2 g IV every 12 hours **OR**
-Cefotaxime (Claforan) 2 g IV every four to six hours **PLUS**
-Vancomycin 15 to 20 mg/kg IV every 8 to 12 hours (not to exceed 2 g per dose or a total daily dose of 60 mg/kg; adjust dose to achieve vancomycin serum trough concentrations of 15 to 20 mcg/mL) PLUS
-In adults >50 years of age: Ampicillin 2 g IV every four hours.

Empiric therapy impaired cell-mediated immunity:
-Vancomycin 15 to 20 mg/kg IV every 8 to 12 hours (not to exceed 2 g per

dose or a total daily dose of 60 mg/kg; adjust dose to achieve vancomycin serum trough concentrations of 15 to 20 mcg/mL **PLUS**
-Ampicillin 2 g IV every four hours **PLUS EITHER**
-Cefepime (Maxipime) 2 g IV every eight hours **OR**
-Meropenem (Merrem) 2 g IV every eight hours.
Fungal Endocarditis:
-Amphotericin B 0.5 mg/kg/d IV plus flucytosine (5-FC) 150 mg/kg/d PO.
9. Symptomatic Medications:
-Famotidine (Pepcid) 20 mg IV/PO q12h.
-Acetaminophen (Tylenol) 325-650 mg PO q4-6h prn temp >39° C.
-Docusate sodium 100-200 mg PO qhs.
10. Extras: CXR PA and LAT, echocardiogram, ECG. Cardiac surgery consult. Infectious diseases consult.
11. Labs: CBC with differential, Basic metabolic panel, basic chemistry. Blood C&S x 3 over 24h, serum bactericidal titers, minimum inhibitory concentration, minimum bactericidal concentration. Repeat C&S in 48h, then once a week. Antibiotic levels peak and trough at 3rd dose. UA, urine C&S.

Pneumonia

1. Admit to:
2. Diagnosis: Pneumonia
3. Condition:
4. Vital Signs: q8h. Call physician if BP >160/90, <90/60; P >120, <50; R>25/min, <10; T >38.5°C or O$_2$ saturation <90%.
5. Activity: Up ad lib, bathroom privileges.
6. Nursing: Pulse oximeter, inputs and outputs, nasotracheal suctioning prn, incentive spirometry.
7. Diet: Regular.
8. IV Fluids: IV D5 ½ NS at 125 cc/hr.
9. Special Medications:
-Oxygen 100% by non-rebreather (reservoir) to maintain O$_2$ saturation >94%.
Non-ICU patients without underlying lung disease with community-acquired pneumonia:
-Ceftriaxone (Rocephin) 1 to 2 g IV daily, cefotaxime (Claforan) 1 to 2 g IV every eight hours, ceftaroline (Teflaro) 600 mg IV every 12 hours, ertapenem (Invanz) 1 g IV daily, or ampicillin-sulbactam (Unasyn) 1.5 to 3 g IV every six hours plus a macrolide (azithromycin (Zithromax) [500 mg IV or orally daily] or clarithromycin XL (Biaxin) [two 500 mg tablets once daily]). Doxycycline (100 mg orally or IV twice daily) may be used as an alternative to a macrolide.
-Monotherapy with a respiratory fluoroquinolone levofloxacin (Levaquin) 750 mg PO or IV daily or moxifloxacin 400 mg PO or IV daily).
-Monotherapy with tigecycline (Tygacil) 100 mg IV once, followed by 50 mg IV every 12 hours is used for patients intolerant of beta-lactams and fluoroquinolones.
-If the patient has risk factors for Pseudomonas or MRSA, coverage for these organisms should be included, as in the following section.
Intensive Care Unit Patients:
-**Pseudomonas aeruginosa or MRSA:** Ceftriaxone (Rocephin) 1 to 2 g daily, cefotaxime (Claforan) 1 to 2 g every eight hours, or

ampicillin-sulbactam (Unasyn) 1.5 to 3 g every six hours) plus
azithromycin 500 mg daily or levofloxacin 750 mg daily or moxifloxacin
400 mg daily.
- **Bronchiectasis or COPD and frequent antimicrobial or glucocorticoid
use:** Pneumococcus, P. aeruginosa, and Legionella spp regimens include
combination therapy with a beta-lactam antibiotic and a fluoroquinolone:
  - Piperacillin-tazobactam (Zosyn) 4.5 g every six hours **OR**
  - Imipenem (Primaxin) 500 mg IV every six hours **OR**
  - Meropenem (Merrem) 1 g every eight hours **OR**
  - Cefepime (Maxipime) 2 g every eight hours **OR**
  - Ceftazidime (Fortaz) 2 g every eight hours
  PLUS
  - Ciprofloxacin (Cipro) 400 mg every eight hours **OR**
  - Levofloxacin (Levaquin) 750 mg daily.
  - Empiric therapy for CA-MRSA should be given to hospitalized patients.
  Vancomycin 15 mg/kg IV every 12 hours, adjusted to a trough level of
  15 to 20 mcg/mL or linezolid 600 mg IV every 12 hours. Clindamycin
  (600 mg IV or orally three times daily) may be used as an alternative
  to vancomycin or linezolid if susceptible. Ceftaroline (Teflaro) is active
  against most strains of MRSA. Linezolid (Zynox) may be given orally
  600 mg PO every 12 hours.
10. **Symptomatic Medications:**
  - Acetaminophen (Tylenol) 650 mg 2 tab PO q4-6h prn temp >38°C or pain.
  - Docusate sodium (Colace) 100 mg PO qhs.
  - Famotidine (Pepcid) 20 mg IV/PO q12h.
  - Heparin 5000 U SQ q12h or pneumatic compression stockings.
11. **Extras:** CXR PA and LAT, ECG, PPD.
12. **Labs:** CBC with differential, Basic metabolic panel, basic chemistry,
  ABG. Blood C&S x 2. Sputum Gram stain, C&S. Methenamine silver
  sputum stain (PCP); AFB smear/culture. Aminoglycoside levels peak and
  trough 3rd dose. UA, urine culture.

Specific Therapy for Pneumonia

Pneumococcus:
- Ceftriaxone (Rocephin) 2 gm IV q12h **OR**
- Cefotaxime (Claforan) 2 gm IV q6h **OR**
- Erythromycin 500 mg IV q6h **OR**
- Levofloxacin (Levaquin) 500 mg IV q24h **OR**
- Vancomycin 1 gm IV q12h if drug resistance.

Staphylococcus aureus:
- Nafcillin 2 gm IV q4h **OR**
- Oxacillin 2 gm IV q4h.

Klebsiella pneumoniae:
- Gentamicin 1.5-2 mg/kg IV, then 1.0-1.5 mg/kg IV q8h or 7 mg/kg in 50
  mL of D5W over 60 min IV q24h **OR**
- Ceftizoxime (Cefizox) 1-2 gm IV q8h **OR**
- Cefotaxime (Claforan) 1-2 gm IV q6h.

Methicillin-resistant staphylococcus aureus (MRSA):
- Vancomycin 1 gm IV q12h.

Vancomycin-Resistant Enterococcus:
- Linezolid (Zyvox) 600 mg IV/PO q12h; active against MRSA as well **OR**
- Quinupristin/dalfopristin (Synercid) 7.5 mg/kg IV q8h (does not cover E

faecalis).

Haemophilus influenzae:
-Ampicillin 1-2 gm IV q6h (beta-lactamase negative) **OR**
-Ampicillin/sulbactam (Unasyn) 1.5-3.0 gm IV q6h **OR**
-Cefuroxime (Zinacef) 1.5 gm IV q8h (beta-lactamase pos) **OR**
-Ceftizoxime (Cefizox) 1-2 gm IV q8h **OR**
-Ciprofloxacin (Cipro) 400 mg IV q12h **OR**
-Ofloxacin (Floxin) 400 mg IV q12h.
-Levofloxacin (Levaquin) 500 mg IV q24h.

Pseudomonas aeruginosa:
-Tobramycin 1.5-2.0 mg/kg IV, then 1.5-2.0 mg/kg IV q8h or 7 mg/kg in 50 mL of D5W over 60 min IV q24h **AND EITHER**
-Piperacillin, ticarcillin, mezlocillin or azlocillin 3 gm IV q4h **OR**
-Cefepime (Maxipime) 2 gm IV q12h.

Enterobacter Aerogenes or Cloacae:
-Gentamicin 2.0 mg/kg IV, then 1.5 mg/kg IV q8h **AND EITHER**
Meropenem (Merrem) 1 gm IV q8h **OR**
Imipenem/cilastatin (Primaxin) 0.5-1.0 gm IV q6h.

Serratia Marcescens:
-Ceftizoxime (Cefizox) 1-2 gm IV q8h **OR**
-Aztreonam (Azactam) 1-2 gm IV q6h **OR**
-Imipenem/cilastatin (Primaxin) 0.5-1.0 gm IV q6h **OR**
-Meropenem (Merrem) 1 gm IV q8h.

Mycoplasma pneumoniae:
-Clarithromycin (Biaxin) 500 mg PO bid **OR**
-Azithromycin (Zithromax) 500 mg PO x 1, then 250 mg PO qd for 4 days **OR**
-Erythromycin 500 mg PO or IV q6h **OR**
-Doxycycline (Vibramycin) 100 mg PO/IV q12h **OR**
-Levofloxacin (Levaquin) 500 mg PO/IV q24h.

Legionella pneumoniae:
-Erythromycin 1.0 gm IV q6h **OR**
-Levofloxacin (Levaquin) 500 mg PO/IV q24h.
-Rifampin 600 mg PO qd may be added to erythromycin or levofloxacin.

Moraxella catarrhalis:
-Trimethoprim/sulfamethoxazole (Bactrim, Septra) one DS tab PO bid or 10 mL IV q12h **OR**
-Ampicillin/sulbactam (Unasyn) 1.5-3 gm IV q6h **OR**
-Cefuroxime (Zinacef) 0.75-1.5 gm IV q8h **OR**
-Erythromycin 500 mg IV q6h **OR**
-Levofloxacin (Levaquin) 500 mg PO/IV q24h.

Anaerobic Pneumonia:
-Penicillin G 2 MU IV q4h **OR**
-Clindamycin (Cleocin) 900 mg IV q8h **OR**
-Metronidazole (Flagyl) 500 mg IV q8h.

Pneumocystis Jirovecii Pneumonia in AIDS

1. **Admit to:**
2. **Diagnosis:** PJP pneumonia
3. **Condition:**
4. **Vital Signs:** q2-6h. Call physician if BP >160/90, <90/60; P >120, <50; R>25/min, <10; T >38.5°C; O_2 sat <90%
5. **Activity:** Bedrest, bedside commode.
6. **Nursing:** Pulse oximeter.
7. **Diet:** Regular, encourage fluids.
8. **IV Fluids:** D5 ½ NS at 125 cc/h.
9. **Special Medications:**

Pneumocystis Carinii Pneumonia:
-Oxygen at 2-4 L/min by mask.
-Oral TMP-SMX — Oral trimethoprim-sulfamethoxazole (TMP-SMX) is administered at a dose of TMP 320 mg plus SMX 1600 mg (two double-strength tablets) every eight hours.
-TMP-dapsone — Oral trimethoprim is administered at a dose of 5 mg/kg (typically rounded to the nearest 100 milligrams) three times daily with dapsone 100 mg daily.
-Oral clindamycin-primaquine — Oral clindamycin - primaquine is administered as clindamycin 450 mg four times daily plus primaquine base 15 mg per day.
-Atovaquone — 750 mg twice daily, taken with food for 21 days [13].
-Trimethoprim/sulfamethoxazole (Bactrim, Septra) IV solution is supplied in a 1:5 ratio of TMP to SMX. Patients should receive a total daily dose of 15 mg of TMP/kg/day (20 mL in 250 mL of D5W IVPB q8h) for 21 days [inj: 80/400 mg per 5 mL].
-Pentamidine (Pentam) 4 mg/kg daily IV for 21 days.
-Clindamycin-primaquine: clindamycin is administered at a dose of 600 mg every eight hours along with oral primaquine base 30 mg daily.
-If severe PCP (PaO_2 <70 mm Hg): Prednisone 40 mg twice daily for five days, followed by 40 mg daily for five days, followed by 20 mg daily for 11 days **OR**
-Methylprednisolone (Solu-Medrol) 30 mg IV q12h for 5 days, then 30 mg IV qd for 5 days, then 15 mg IV qd for 11 days.

Pneumocystis Jirovecii Prophylaxis (previous PJP, CD4 <200, or oropharyngeal candidiasis):
-Trimethoprim/SMX DS 160/800 mg PO qd **OR**
-Dapsone (DDS) 50 mg PO bid or 100 mg twice a week; contraindicated in G-6-PD deficiency **OR**
-Atovaquone (Mepron) suspension 1500 mg daily.

10. **Symptomatic Medications:**
-Acetaminophen (Tylenol) 325-650 mg PO q4-6h prn headache or fever.
-Docusate sodium 100-200 mg PO qhs.
10. **Extras:** CXR PA and LAT.
11. **Labs:** Immunofluorescent staining of specimens obtained by sputum induction. PCR test for PJP. Blood 1,3 beta-Dglucan. ABG, CBC, Basic metabolic panel, basic chemistry. Blood C&S x 2. Sputum for Gram stain, C&S, AFB. CD4 count, HIV RNA, VDRL, serum cryptococcal antigen, UA.

HIV Antiretroviral Therapy

HHS Guidelines:

A non-nucleoside reverse transcriptase inhibitor (NNRTI), efavirenz , plus two nucleoside reverse transcriptase inhibitors (NRTIs) **OR**

A boosted protease inhibitor (PI): atazanavir - ritonavir once daily or darunavir -ritonavir once daily plus two NRTIs **OR**

Raltegravir (Isentress) 400 mg twice daily (an integrase inhibitor) with two NRTIs (tenofovir-emtricitabine).

Protease Inhibitors

Atazanavir (Reyataz) 400 mg (two 200 mg capsules) once a day unboosted, and atazanavir 300 mg (one 300 mg capsule) once a day plus ritonavir 100 mg once a day (ie, boosted atazanavir).

Darunavir (Prezista) 800 mg once daily (given as two 400 mg tablets) plus ritonavir (100 mg) once daily.

Non-nucleoside Reverse Transcriptase Inhibitors

Efavirenz (Sustiva) 600 mg once daily.

Integrase Strand Transfer Inhibitors

Raltegravir (Isentress) 400 mg twice daily.

Nucleoside Analogs

Tenofovir-emtricitabine (Truvada) one tablet daily with or without regard to food.

Postexposure HIV Prophylaxis

A. For HCP with a percutaneous, mucous membrane, or nonintact skin exposure to potentially infectious body fluids from a patient with known HIV infection, postexposure prophylaxis (PEP) is provided.

B. The injury should be immediately washed with soap and water.

C. Postexporure prophylaxis consists of tenofovir-emtricitabine (Truvada), one tablet daily, combined with raltegravir, 400 mg twice daily, for four weeks.

Opportunistic Infections in HIV-Infected Patients

Oral Candidiasis:

-Fluconazole (Diflucan) 100-200 mg PO qd **OR**

-Ketoconazole (Nizoral) 400 mg PO qd **OR**

-Itraconazole (Sporanox) 200 mg PO qd **OR**

-Clotrimazole (Mycelex) troches 10 mg dissolved slowly in mouth 5 times/d.

Candida Esophagitis:

-Fluconazole (Diflucan) 200-400 mg PO qd for 14-21 days **OR**

-Ketoconazole (Nizoral) 200 mg PO bid **OR**

-Itraconazole (Sporanox) 200 mg PO qd for 2 weeks.

-Caspofungin (Cancidas) 50 mg IV qd x 2 weeks.

Primary or Recurrent Mucocutaneous HSV

-Acyclovir (Zovirax), 200-400 mg PO 5 times a day for 10 days, or 5 mg/kg IV q8h **OR** in cases of acyclovir resistance, foscarnet, 40 mg/kg IV q8h for 21 days.

Herpes Simplex Encephalitis (or visceral disease):

-Acyclovir (Zovirax) 10 mg/kg IV q8h for 10-21 days.

Herpes Varicella Zoster

-Famciclovir (Famvir) 500 mg PO q8h for 7 days [500 mg] **OR**
-Valacyclovir (Valtrex) 1000 mg PO q8h for 7 days [500 mg] **OR**
-Foscarnet (Foscavir) 40 mg/kg IV q8h **OR**
-Acyclovir (Zovirax) 10 mg/kg IV over 60 min q8h for 7-14 days OR 80 mg PO 5 times/d for 7-10 days.

Cytomegalovirus Retinitis:
-Valganciclovir (Valcyte) PO 900 mg twice daily for 21 days.
-Sight-threatening lesions: Intravitreal injection or implant) or intravenous ganciclovir with oral valganciclovir 900 mg twice daily for 21 days.

Suppressive Treatment for Cytomegalovirus Retinitis:
-Valganciclovir (Valcyte) 900 mg daily.

Acute Toxoplasmosis:
-Pyrimethamine 200 mg, then 50-75 mg qd, plus sulfadiazine 1.0-1.5 gr PO q6h, plus folinic acid 10 mg PO qd **OR**
-Atovaquone (Mepron) 750 mg PO tid.

Suppressive Treatment for Toxoplasmosis:
-Pyrimethamine 25-50 mg PO qd plus sulfadiazine 0.5-1.0 gm PO q6 plus folinic acid 5 mg PO qd **OR**
-Pyrimethamine 50 mg PO qd, plus clindamycin 300 mg PO qid, plus folinic acid 5 mg PO qd.

Cryptococcus Neoformans Meningitis:
-Amphotericin B 0.7-1.0 mg/kg/d IV; total dosage of 2 g, with or without 5 flucytosine 100 mg/kg PO qd in divided doses, followed by fluconazole (Diflucan) 400 mg PO qd or itraconazole (Sporanox) 200 mg PO bid 6 8 weeks **OR**
-Amphotericin B liposomal (Abelcet) 5 mg/kg IV q24h **OR**
-Fluconazole (Diflucan) 400-800 mg PO qd for 8-12 weeks

Suppressive Treatment of Cryptococcus:
-Fluconazole (Diflucan) 200 mg PO qd indefinitely.

Active Tuberculosis:
-Isoniazid (INH) 300 mg PO qd; and rifampin 600 mg PO qd; and pyrazinamide 15-25 mg/kg PO qd (500 mg bid-tid); and ethambutol 15 25 mg/kg PO qd (400 mg bid-tid).
-All four drugs are continued for 2 months; isoniazid and rifampin are continued for a period of at least 9 months and at least 6 months after the last negative cultures.
-Pyridoxine (Vitamin B6) 50 mg PO qd concurrent with INH.

Prophylaxis for Latent Tuberculosis:
- Isoniazid 900 mg plus rifapentine 900 mg given as directly observed doses together once weekly for 12 weeks

Disseminated Mycobacterium Avium Complex (MAC):
-Clarithromycin (Biaxin) 500 mg PO bid **AND**
Ethambutol 800-1000 mg PO qd; with or without rifabutin 450 mg qd.

Prophylaxis against Mycobacterium Avium Complex:
-Azithromycin (Zithromax) 1200 mg once a week.

Disseminated Coccidioidomycosis:
-Amphotericin (Fungizone) B 0.5-0.8 mg/kg IV qd, to a total dose 2.0 gm **OR**
-Amphotericin B liposomal (Abelcet) 5 mg/kg IV q24h **OR**
-Fluconazole (Diflucan) 400-800 mg PO or IV qd.

Disseminated Histoplasmosis:
-Amphotericin B (Fungizone) 0.5-0.8 mg/kg IV qd, to a total dose 15 mg/kg **OR**
-Amphotericin B liposomal (Abelcet) 5 mg/kg IV q24h **OR**

-Fluconazole (Diflucan) 400 mg PO qd **OR**
-Itraconazole (Sporanox) 300 mg PO bid for 3 days, then 200 mg PO bid.
Suppressive Treatment for Histoplasmosis:
  -Fluconazole (Diflucan) 400 mg PO qd **OR**
  -Itraconazole (Sporanox) 200 mg PO bid.

Septic Arthritis

1. **Admit to:**
2. **Diagnosis:** Septic arthritis
3. **Condition:**
4. **Vital Signs:** q shift
5. **Activity:** Up in chair as tolerated. Bedside commode with assistance.
6. **Nursing:** Warm compresses prn, keep joint immobilized. Passive range of motion exercises of the affected joint bid.
7. **Diet:** Regular diet.
8. **IV Fluids:** Saline lock
9. **Special Medications:**

If the Gram stain of the synovial fluid shows gram-positive cocci:
  -Vancomycin 30 mg/kg daily IV in two divided doses, not to exceed 2 g per day.

If the Gram stain of the synovial fluid shows gram-negative bacilli:
  -Ceftazidime 1 to 2 g IV every eight hours or
  -Ceftriaxone 2 g IV once daily) or
  -Cefotaxime 2 g IV every eight hours
  -Ceftazidime should be given with gentamicin 3 to 5 mg/kg per day in 32 or 3 divided doses when Pseudomonas aeruginosa is considered to be a likely pathogen (eg, in patients who inject illicit drugs).
  -In cephalosporin-allergic patients, treat with ciprofloxacin 400 mg IV every12 hours or 500 to 750 mg orally twice daily.
  -If the initial Gram stain is negative, treat with vancomycin in the immunocompetent patient and with vancomycin plus a third generation cephalosporin in the immunocompromised patient, in injection drug users or in traumatic bacterial arthritis.

10. **Symptomatic Medications:**
  -Hydrocodone/acetaminophen (Vicodin), 1-2 tab q4-6h PO prn pain.
  -Acetaminophen and codeine (Tylenol 3) 1-2 PO q4-6h prn pain.
  -Heparin 5000 U SQ bid.
  -Famotidine (Pepcid) 20 mg IV/PO q12h.
  -Zolpidem (Ambien) 5-10 mg qhs prn insomnia.
  -Docusate sodium 100-200 mg PO qhs.
11. **Extras:** X-ray views of joint (AP and lateral), CXR. Synovial fluid culture. Physical therapy exercise program.
12. **Labs:** CBC, basic metabolic panel, basic chemistry, blood C&S x 2, VDRL, UA. Gonorrhea cultures of urethra, cervix. Antibiotic levels. Blood cultures x 2 for gonorrhea.
Synovial fluid:
  Tube 1 - Glucose, protein, lactate, pH.
  Tube 2 - Gram stain, C&S.
  Tube 3 - Cell count.

Septic Shock

1. **Admit to:**
2. **Diagnosis:** Sepsis
3. **Condition:**
4. **Vital Signs:** q1h; Call physician if BP >160/90, <90/60; P >120, <50; R>25/min, <10; T >38.5°C; urine output < 25 cc/hr for 4h, O_2 saturation <90%.
5. **Activity:** Bed rest.
6. **Nursing:** Inputs and outputs, pulse oximeter. Foley catheter to closed drainage.
7. **Diet:** NPO
8. **IV Fluids:** 1 liter of normal saline wide open, then D5 ½ NS at 125 cc/h
9. **Special Medications:**
   -Oxygen at 2-5 L/min by NC or mask.

Antibiotic Therapy
   -Vancomycin 1 gm q12h with one of the following:
   -Ceftriaxone 2 g IV once daily; or cefotaxime 2 g IV q8h **OR**
   -Piperacillin-tazobactam (Zosyn) 3.375-4.5 gm IV q6h.
   -Imipenem (Primaxin) 0.5-1.0 gm IV q6h
   -If Pseudomonas is a possible pathogen, combine vancomycin with two of the following: Ceftazidime 2 g IV every eight hours, cefepime 2 gm IV q12h, or
   -Antipseudomonal carbapenem (eg, imipenem (Primaxin) 1.0 gm IV q6h meropenem (Merrem) 0.5-1.0 gm IV q8h), or
   -Antipseudomonal beta-lactam/beta-lactamase inhibitor (eg piperacillin-tazobactam), or
   -Anti-pseudomonal fluoroquinolone (eg, ciprofloxacin 400 mg IV every12 hours), **OR**
   -Gentamicin 7 mg/kg in 50 mL of D5W over 60 min IV q24h **OR**
   -Aztreonam (Azactam) 1-2 gm IV q6-8h; max 8 g/day.)

Additional Therapies
   -Severe septic shock with systolic blood pressure <90 mmHg: Intravenous hydrocortisone 50 mg IV q6hor for five to seven days.

Blood Pressure Support
   -Dopamine 4-20 mcg/kg/min (400 mg in 250 cc D5W, 1600 mcg/mL).
   -Norepinephrine 2-8 mcg/min IV infusion (8 mg in 250 mL D5W).
   -Dobutamine 5 mcg/kg/min, and titrate blood pressure to keep systolic BP >90 mm Hg; max 10 mcg/kg/min.

10. **Symptomatic Medications:**
    -Acetaminophen (Tylenol) 650 mg PR q4-6h prn temp >39°C.
    -Famotidine (Pepcid) 20 mg IV/PO q12h.
    -Heparin 5000 U SQ q12h or pneumatic compression stockings.
    -Docusate sodium 100-200 mg PO qhs.
11. **Extras:** CXR, KUB, ECG. Ultrasound, lumbar puncture.
12. **Labs:** CBC with differential, basic metabolic panel, basic chemistry, blood C&S x 3, T&C for 3-6 units PRBC, INR/PTT, drug levels peak and trough at 3rd dose. UA. Cultures of urine, sputum, wound, IV catheters, decubitus ulcers, pleural fluid.

Peritonitis

- **Admit to:**
- **Diagnosis:** Peritonitis
- **Condition:**
- **Vital Signs:** q8h. Call physician if BP >160/90, <90/60; P >120, <50; R>25/min, <10; T >38.5°C.
- **Activity:** Bed rest.
- **Nursing:** Guaiac stools.
- **Diet:** NPO
- **IV Fluids:** D5 ½ NS at 125 cc/h.
- **Special Medications:**

Primary Bacterial Peritonitis:

-Cefotaxime (Claforan) for five days. Treatment is discontinued if there has been the usual dramatic response.

-Intravenous albumin 1.5 g/kg within six hours of diagnosis and 1.0 g/kg on day 3. Albumin should be given if the creatinine is >1 mg/dL, the blood urea nitrogen is >30 mg/dL, or the total bilirubin is >4 mg/dL.

Prophylaxis:

-Norfloxacin (Noroxin) 400 mg/day, or trimethoprim-sulfamethoxazole therapy (one double-strength tablet once daily) in patients who have had one or more episodes of SBP.

-Prolonged prophylaxis is recommended for patients with cirrhosis and ascitic fluid total protein <1.5 g/dL with at least one of the following: (a) Child-Pugh ≥9 points and serum bilirubin ≥3 mg/dL or (b) serum creatinine ≥1.2 mg/dL or blood urea nitrogen ≥25 mg/dL or serum sodium ≤130 meq/L.

-In patients with cirrhosis who are hospitalized for gastrointestinal bleeding: Initial intravenous ceftriaxone 1 g daily. Transition patients to 400 mg of norfloxacin orally twice daily or trimethoprim-sulfamethoxazole (one double-strength tablet twice daily) for seven days of total antibiotic use once bleeding has been controlled.

-Patients with cirrhosis hospitalized for other reasons who have an ascitic fluid protein concentration <1 g/dL should be treated with norfloxacin (400 mg/day) or trimethoprim-sulfamethoxazole until the time of discharge.

Empiric initial therapy for peritonitis in continuous peritoneal dialysis:

-Gram positive organisms may be covered by vancomycin 1 gm q12h (1 gm in 250 cc D5W over 60 min).

-Gram negative organisms may be covered by a third-generation cephalosporin or an aminoglycoside.

Secondary Bacterial Peritonitis – Abdominal Perforation or Rupture:
Option 1:

-Ampicillin 1-2 gm IV q4-6h **AND**

Gentamicin or tobramycin 7 mg/kg in 50 mL of D5W over 60 min IV q24h, **AND**

Metronidazole (Flagyl) 500 mg IV q8h **OR**

Cefoxitin (Mefoxin) 1-2 gm IV q6h **OR**

Cefotetan (Cefotan) 1-2 gm IV q12h.

Option 2:

-Ticarcillin/clavulanate (Timentin) 3.1 gm IV q4-6h (200-300 mg/kg/d) with an aminoglycoside as above **OR**

-Piperacillin/tazobactam (Zosyn) 3.375 gm IV q6h with an aminoglycosid as above **OR**
-Ampicillin/sulbactam (Unasyn) 1.5-3.0 gm IV q6h with aminoglycosid as above **OR**
-Imipenem/cilastatin (Primaxin) 0.5-1.0 gm IV q6-8h **OR**
-Meropenem (Merrem) 500-1000 mg IV q8h.

Fungal Peritonitis:
-Amphotericin B peritoneal dialysis, 2 mg/L of dialysis fluid over the firs 24 hours, then 1.5 mg in each liter **OR**
-Fluconazole (Diflucan) 200 mg IV x 1, then 100 mg IV qd.
-Caspofungin (Candidas) 70 mg IV x1, then 50 mg IV qd.

10. **Symptomatic Medications:**
-Famotidine (Pepcid) 20 mg IV/PO q12h.
-Acetaminophen (Tylenol) 325 mg PO/PR q4-6h prn temp >38.5°C.
-Heparin 5000 U SQ q12h.

11. **Extras:** Plain film, upright abdomen, lateral decubitus, CXR PA and LAT surgery consult; ECG, abdominal ultrasound, CT scan.

12. **Labs:** CBC with differential, basic metabolic panel, basic chemistry amylase, lactate, INR/PTT, UA with micro, C&S; drug levels peak an trough 3rd dose.

Paracentesis Tube 1: Cell count and differential (1-2 mL, EDTA purple to tube).

Tube 2: Gram stain of sediment; inject 10-20 mL into anaerobic and aerobi culture bottle; AFB, fungal C&S (3-4 mL).

Tube 3: Glucose, protein, albumin, LDH, triglycerides, specific gravity, biliru bin, amylase (2-3 mL, red top tube).

Syringe: pH, lactate (3 mL).

Diverticulitis

1. **Admit to:**
2. **Diagnosis:** Diverticulitis
3. **Condition:**
4. **Vital Signs:** qid. Call physician if BP systolic >160/90, <90/60; P >120 <50; R>25/min, <10; T >38.5°C.
5. **Activity:** Up ad lib.
6. **Nursing:** Inputs and outputs.
7. **Diet:** NPO. Advance to clear liquids as tolerated.
8. **IV Fluids:** 0.5-2 L NS over 1-2 hr then, D5 ½ NS at 125 cc/hr. NG tube at low intermittent suction (if obstructed).
9. **Special Medications:**
-Ciprofloxacin (Cipro) 500 mg PO twice daily plus metronidazole (500 mg PO three times daily) for 10 to 14 days **OR**
-Amoxicillin-clavulanate (Augmentin) 875/125 mg twice daily for 10 to 14 days is an acceptable alternative.
-For complicated diverticulitis , intravenous antibiotics are administered until the inflammation is stabilized and pain and tenderness are resolving. The patient is then transitioned to oral antibiotics for a 10 to 14 day course.
-Ampicillin-sulbactam (Unasyn) 3 g every six hours **OR**
-Piperacillin /tazobactam (Zosyn) 3.375 g IV q6h **OR**
-Ticarcillin-clavulanate (3.1 g every six hours) **OR**
-Ceftriaxone (1 g IV every 24 hours) **PLUS**

-Metronidazole (Flagyl) 500 mg IV every 8 hours.

or patients with beta-lactam intolerance, alternative empiric regimens include:

-Ciprofloxacin (Cipro) 400 mg IV every 12 hours or

-Levofloxacin (Levaquin) 500 mg or 750 IV daily) **PLUS** metronidazole (Flagyl) 500 mg IV every 8 hours) OR

-Imipenem (500 mg every six hours) **OR**

-Meropenem (Merrem) 1 g every eight hours **OR**

-Ertapenem (Invanz) 1 g daily.

0. Symptomatic Medications:

-Morphine sulfate 5-10 mg IV/IM q2-4h prn pain

-Zolpidem (Ambien) 5-10 mg qhs PO prn insomnia

1. Extras: Acute abdomen series, CXR PA and LAT, ECG, CT scan of abdomen, ultrasound, surgery and GI consults.

2. Labs: CBC with differential, basic metabolic panel, basic chemistry, albumen, amylase, lipase, blood cultures x 2, drug levels peak and trough 3rd dose. UA, C&S.

ower Urinary Tract Infection

. **Admit to:**

. **Diagnosis:** UTI.

. **Condition:**

. **Vital Signs:** q shift. Call physician if BP <90/60; >160/90; R >30, <10; P >120, <50; T >38.5°C.

. **Activity:** Up ad lib

. **Nursing:**

. **Diet:** Regular

. **IV Fluids:** Saline lock with flush q shift.

. **Special Medications:**

ower Urinary Tract Infection (treat for 3-7 days):

ystitis in Women:

Nitrofurantoin monohydrate/macrocrystals (Macrobid) 100 mg orally twice daily for 5 days.

Trimethoprim-sulfamethoxazole one double strength tablet [160/800 mg] twice daily for 3 days.

Fosfomycin (Monurol) 3 grams single dose.

yelonephritis in Women and Men:

utpatient

iprofloxacin (Cipro) 500 mg orally twice daily for seven days or 1000 mg extended release once daily for seven days or levofloxacin (Levoquin) 750 mg orally once daily for five to seven days with ceftriaxone 1 gram IV or a 24-hour dose of gentamicin 7 mg/kg.

rimethoprim-sulfamethoxazole (160/800 mg [one double-strength tablet] twice-daily) or an oral beta-lactam, if the uropathogen is susceptible. Ceftriaxone or gentamicin 7 mg/kg. Patients with hypersensitivity and/or resistance may be treated with aztreonam 1 g IV every 8 to 12 hours.

ipatient:

-Ciprofloxacin (Cipro) 250 mg IV q12h or levofloxacin (Levaquin) 500 mg IV/PO q24h. IV, an aminoglycoside (with ampicillin), an ex-tended-spectrum cephalosporin, an extended-spectrum penicillin, or a carbapenem.

-Trimethoprim-sulfamethoxazole (Septra) 1 double strength tab (160/800

mg) PO bid.
-Norfloxacin (Noroxin) 400 mg PO bid.
-Lomefloxacin (Maxaquin) 400 mg PO qd.
-Enoxacin (Penetrex) 200-400 mg PO q12h; 1h before or 2h after meals
-Cefpodoxime (Vantin) 100 mg PO bid.
-Cephalexin (Keflex) 500 mg PO q6h.
-Cefixime (Suprax) 200 mg PO q12h or 400 mg PO qd.
-Cefazolin (Ancef) 1-2 gm IV q8h.

Prophylaxis (≥3 episodes/yr):
-Trimethoprim/SMX single strength tab PO qhs.

Cystitis in Men:
TMP-SMX is one double strength tablet [160/800 mg] twice daily for 7-1
days.
Ciprofloxacin (Cipro) 500 mg orally twice daily or 1000 mg extended release
once daily for 7-14 days.
Levofloxacin (Levoquin) 500 to 750 mg orally once daily for 7-14 days.

Candida Cystitis
-Fluconazole (Diflucan) 100 mg PO or IV x 1 dose, then 50 mg PO or IV
qd for 5 days **OR**
-Amphotericin B continuous bladder irrigation, 50 mg/1000 mL sterile
water via 3-way. Foley catheter at 1 L/d for 5 days.

10. Symptomatic Medications:
-Phenazopyridine (Pyridium) 100 mg PO tid.
-Docusate sodium (Colace) 100 mg PO qhs.
-Acetaminophen (Tylenol) 325-650 mg PO q4-6h prn temp >39° C.
-Zolpidem (Ambien) 5-10 mg qhs prn insomnia.

11. Extras: Renal ultrasound.

12. Labs: CBC, basic metabolic panel. UA with micro, urine Gram stain
C&S.

Pyelonephritis

1. Admit to:
2. Diagnosis: Pyelonephritis
3. Condition:
4. Vital Signs: tid. Call physician if BP <90/60; >160/90; R >30, <10; P
>120, <50; T >38.5°C.
5. Activity:
6. Nursing: Inputs and outputs.
7. Diet: Regular
8. IV Fluids: D5 ½ NS at 125 cc/h.
9. Special Medications:
-Trimethoprim-sulfamethoxazole (Septra) 160/800 mg (10 mL in 100 ml
D5W IV over 2 hours) q12h or 1 double strength tab PO bid.
-Ciprofloxacin (Cipro) 500 mg PO bid or 400 mg IV q12h.
-Norfloxacin (Noroxin) 400 mg PO bid.
-Ofloxacin (Floxin) 400 mg PO or IV bid.
-Levofloxacin (Levaquin) 500 mg PO/IV q24h.
-In more severely ill patients, treatment with an IV third-generation
cephalosporin, or ticarcillin/clavulanic acid, or piperacillin/tazobactam
or imipenem is recommended with an aminoglycoside.
-Ceftizoxime (Cefizox) 1 gm IV q8h.
-Ceftazidime (Fortaz) 1 gm IV q8h.

-Ticarcillin/clavulanate (Timentin) 3.1 gm IV q6h.
-Piperacillin/tazobactam (Zosyn) 3.375 gm IV/PB q6h.
-Imipenem/cilastatin (Primaxin) 0.5-1.0 gm IV q6-8h.
-Gentamicin or tobramycin, 2 mg/kg IV, then 1.5 mg/kg q8h or 7 mg/kg in 50 mL of D5W over 60 min IV q24h.

10. Symptomatic Medications:
-Phenazopyridine (Pyridium) 100 mg PO tid.
-Morphine sulfate 5-10 mg IV/IM q2-4h prn pain
-Docusate sodium (Colace) 100 mg PO qhs.
-Acetaminophen (Tylenol) 325-650 mg PO q4-6h prn temp >39° C.
-Zolpidem (Ambien) 5-10 mg qhs prn insomnia.

11. Extras: Renal ultrasound, KUB.

12. Labs: CBC with differential, basic metabolic panel. UA with micro, urine Gram stain, C&S; blood C&S x 2. Drug levels peak and trough third dose.

Osteomyelitis

1. Admit to:

2. Diagnosis: Osteomyelitis

3. Condition:

4. Vital Signs: qid. Call physician if BP <90/60; T >38.5°C.

5. Activity: Bed rest with bathroom privileges.

6. Nursing: Keep involved extremity elevated. Range of motion exercises tid.

7. Diet: Regular, high fiber.

8. IV Fluids: Saline lock with flush q shift.

9. Special Medications:

Empiric Therapy:
-Vancomycin 30 mg/kg per 24 hours in two equally divided doses.

Gram-negative organisms:
-Ciprofloxacin (Cipro) 400 mg IV every 8 hours or 12 hours.

MSSA:
-Penicillin (4 million units every four hours), if susceptible
-Nafcillin 2 g every four hours **OR**
-Flucloxacillin (Floxapen) 2 g q6h **OR**
-Cefazolin (Ancef) 2 g q8h.

MRSA:
-Vancomycin 30 mg/kg per 24 hours in two equally divided doses **OR**
-Daptomycin (Cubicin) 6 mg/kg/day.
-Trimethoprim-sulfamethoxazole (4 mg/kg/dose of the trimethoprim) in combination with rifampin 600 mg qd, linezolid (600 mg PO or IV bid), or clindamycin 600 mg PO or IV tid.

Pseudomonas aeruginosa following nail puncture:
-Ceftazidime (Fortaz) 2 g IV every eight hours.
-Ciprofloxacin (Cipro) 400 mg IV every 8 hours or 12 hours OR
-Aztreonam (Aztactam) 2 g IV q8h, or imipenem 500 mg IV q6h plus (tobramycin or gentamicin [3 to 5 mg/kg per day IV divided bid-tid] or amikacin [7.5 mg/kg IV every 12 hours]). Oral ciprofloxacin (750 mg bid).

10. Symptomatic Medications:
-Morphine sulfate 5-10 mg IV/IM q2-4h prn pain
-Docusate (Colace) 100 mg PO qhs.
-Heparin 5000 U SQ bid.

11. **Extras:** Technetium/gallium bone scans, multiple X-ray views, CT/MR scan. Hyperbaric oxygen (HBO) and negative pressure wound therapy (NPWT). Surgical consult, infectious disease consult.
12. **Labs:** CBC with differential, basic metabolic panel, blood C&S x 3, MIC, MBC, ESR,, C-reactive protein, UA with micro, C&S. Needle biopsy of bone for C&S. Trough antibiotic levels.

Active Pulmonary Tuberculosis

1. **Admit to:**
2. **Diagnosis:** Active Pulmonary Tuberculosis
3. **Condition:**
4. **Vital Signs:** q shift
5. **Activity:** Up ad lib in room.
6. **Nursing:** Respiratory isolation.
7. **Diet:** Regular
8. **Special Medications:**

Initial phase: Four drugs (isoniazid [INH], rifampin [RIF], pyrazinamide [PZA], and ethambutol [EMB]) are used in the initial phase of previously untreated tuberculosis for two months: Daily for two weeks, then twice weekly for six weeks schedule facilitates administration of DOT.

Continuation phase of treatment for pulmonary tuberculosis is administered for four or seven months and consists of INH and RIF. Most patients are treated with a four-month (total duration of treatment six months).
  -Isoniazid 300 mg PO qd (5 mg/kg/d, max 300 mg/d) **AND**
   Rifampin 600 mg PO qd (10 mg/kg/d, 600 mg/d max) **AND**
   Pyrazinamide 500 mg PO bid-tid (15-30 mg/kg/d, max 2.5 gm) **AND**
   Ethambutol 400 mg PO bid-tid (15-25 mg/kg/d, 2.5 gm/d max).
  -Pyridoxine 50 mg PO qd with INH.

Prophylaxis
  -Isoniazid 300 mg PO qd (5 mg/kg/d) x 6-9 months.
9. **Extras:** CXR PA, LAT, ECG.
10. **Labs:** CBC with differential, SMA7 and 12, LFTs, HIV serology. First AM sputum for AFB x 3 samples.

Cellulitis

1. **Admit to:**
2. **Diagnosis:** Cellulitis
3. **Condition:**
4. **Vital Signs:** tid. Call physician if BP <90/60; T >38.5°C
5. **Activity:** Up ad lib.
6. **Nursing:** Keep affected extremity elevated; warm compresses prn.
7. **Diet:** Regular, encourage fluids.
8. **IV Fluids:** Saline lock with flush q shift.
9. **Special Medications:**

Empiric Therapy for Cellulitis
  -Nafcillin or oxacillin 1-2 gm IV q4-6h **OR**
  -Cefazolin (Ancef) 1-2 gm IV q8h **OR**
  -Vancomycin 1 gm q12h (1 gm in 250 cc D5W over 1h) **OR**
  -Dicloxacillin 500 mg PO qid; may add penicillin VK, 500 mg PO qid, to

increase coverage for streptococcus **OR**
-Cephalexin (Keflex) 500 mg PO qid.

Immunosuppressed, Diabetic Patients, or Ulcerated Lesions:
-Nafcillin or cefazolin and gentamicin or aztreonam. Add clindamycin or metronidazole if septic.
-Cefazolin (Ancef) 1-2 gm IV q8h.
-Cefoxitin (Mefoxin) 1-2 gm IV q6-8h.
-Gentamicin 2 mg/kg, then 1.5 mg/kg IV q8h or 7 mg/kg in 50 mL of D5W over 60 min IV q24h **OR** aztreonam (Azactam) 1-2 gm IV q6h **PLUS**
-Metronidazole (Flagyl) 500 mg IV q8h or clindamycin 900 mg IV q8h.
-Ticarcillin/clavulanate (Timentin) **(single-drug treatment)** 3.1 gm IV q4-6h.
-Ampicillin/Sulbactam (Unasyn) **(single-drug therapy)** 1.5-3.0 gm IV q6h.
-Imipenem/cilastatin (Primaxin) **(single-drug therapy)** 0.5-1 gm IV q6-8h.

10. **Symptomatic Medications:**
-Acetaminophen/codeine (Tylenol #3) 1-2 PO q4-6h prn pain.
-Docusate (Colace) 100 mg PO qhs.
-Acetaminophen (Tylenol) 325-650 mg PO q4-6h prn temp >39° C.
-Zolpidem (Ambien) 5-10 mg qhs prn insomnia.
11. **Extras:** X-ray views of site, technetium/Gallium scans.
12. **Labs:** CBC, basic metabolic panel, blood C&S x 2. Leading edge aspirate for Gram stain, C&S; UA, antibiotic levels.

Pelvic Inflammatory Disease

1. **Admit to:**
2. **Diagnosis:** Pelvic Inflammatory Disease
3. **Condition:**
4. **Vital Signs:** q8h. Call physician if BP >160/90, <90/60; P >120, <50; R>25/min, <10; T >38.5°C
5. **Activity:** Up ad lib.
6. **Nursing:** Inputs and outputs.
7. **Diet:** Regular
8. **IV Fluids:** D5 ½ NS at 100-125 cc/hr.
9. **Special Medications:**
-Ceftriaxone (Rocephin) 250 mg IM; and doxycycline (100 mg orally twice daily) and metronidazole for 14 days **OR**
-Cefoxitin (Mefoxin) 2 g intravenously every 6 hours or cefotetan 2 g IV every 12 hours) and doxycycline (100 mg orally every 12 hours). Continue doxycycline 100 mg twice daily alone for 14 days **OR**
-Clindamycin (900 mg intravenously every eight hours) plus gentamicin (2 mg/kg loading dose followed by a 1.5 mg/kg every eight hours). Single daily intravenous dosing of gentamicin may be substituted for three times daily dosing. Continue doxycycline 100 mg twice daily alone after 24 hours of sustained clinical improvement.
-**Severe penicillin allergy:** Levofloxacin 500 mg orally once daily for 14 days AND a single dose of azithromycin (2 grams orally).
10. **Symptomatic Medications:**
-Acetaminophen (Tylenol) 1-2 tabs PO q4-6h prn pain or temperature >38.5°C.
-Morphine sulfate 5-10 mg IV/IM q2-4h prn pain
-Zolpidem (Ambien) 10 mg PO qhs prn insomnia.
11. **Labs:** beta-HCG, CBC, basic metabolic panel, basic chemistry. GC

NAAT, chlamydia NAAT. UA with micro, C&S, VDRL, HIV, blood cultures x 2. Pelvic ultrasound.

Gastrointestinal Disorders

Gastroesophageal Reflux Disease

1. **Admit to:**
2. **Diagnosis:** Gastroesophageal reflux disease.
3. **Condition:**
4. **Vital Signs:** q4h. Call physician if BP >160/90, <90/60; P >120, <50; T >38.5°C.
5. **Activity:** Up ad lib. Elevate the head of the bed with blocks by 6 inches.
6. **Nursing:** Guaiac stools.
7. **Diet:** Low-fat diet; no colas, chocolate, citrus juices; avoid supine position after meals; no eating within 3 hours of bedtime.
8. **IV Fluids:** Saline lock with flush q shift.
9. **Special Medications:**
   -Omeprazole (Prilosec) 20 mg PO bid (30 minutes prior to meals) **OR**
   -Pantoprazole (Protonix) 40 mg PO/IV q24h **OR**
   -Nizatidine (Axid) 300 mg PO qhs **OR**
   -Lansoprazole (Prevacid) 15-30 mg PO qd [15, 30 mg caps] **OR**
   -Esomeprazole (Nexium) 20 or 40 mg PO qd **OR**
   -Rabeprazole (Aciphex) 20 mg delayed-release tablet PO qd.
   -Ranitidine (Zantac) 50 mg IV bolus, then continuous infusion at 12.5 mg/h (300 mg in 250 mL D5W at 11 mL/h over 24h) or 50 mg IV q8h **OR**
   -Cimetidine (Tagamet) 300 mg IV bolus, then continuous infusion at 50 mg/h (1200 mg in 250 mL D5W over 24h) or 300 mg IV q6-8h **OR**
   -Famotidine (Pepcid) 20 mg IV q12h.
10. **Symptomatic Medications:**
    -Mylanta Plus or Maalox Plus 30 mg PO q2h prn.
    -Trimethobenzamide (Tigan) 100-250 mg PO or 100-200 mg IM/PR q6h prn nausea **OR**
    -Ondansetron (Zofran) 2-4 mg IV q4h or 8 mg PO q8h prn nausea or vomiting. **OR**
    -Prochlorperazine (Compazine) 5-10 mg IM/IV/PO/PR q4-6h or 25 mg PR q4-6h prn nausea.
11. **Extras:** Upright abdomen, KUB, CXR, ECG, endoscopy. GI consult, surgery consult.
12. **Labs:** CBC, basic metabolic panel, basic chemistry, amylase, lipase, LDH. UA.

Peptic Ulcer Disease

1. **Admit to:**
2. **Diagnosis:** Peptic ulcer disease.
3. **Condition:**
4. **Vital Signs:** q4h. Call physician if BP >160/90, <90/60; P >120, <50; T >38.5°C.
5. **Activity:** Up ad lib
6. **Nursing:** Guaiac stools.
7. **Diet:** NPO 48h, then regular diet.
8. **IV Fluids:** D5 ½ NS with 20 mEq KCL at 125 cc/h. NG tube at low intermittent suction (if obstructed).
9. **Special Medications:**
   -Esomeprazole (NexIUM) 20 mg or 40 mg IV or PO once daily.
   -Pantoprazole (Protonix) 40 mg PO/IV q24h **OR**
   -Nizatidine (Axid) 300 mg PO qhs **OR**
   -Omeprazole (Prilosec) 20 mg PO bid (30 minutes prior to meals) **OR**
   -Lansoprazole (Prevacid) 15-30 mg PO qd prior to breakfast [15, 30 mg caps]. **OR**
   -Rabeprazole (Aciphex) 20 mg delayed-release tablet PO qd.
   -Dexlansoprazole (Dexilant) 60 mg once daily for up to 8 weeks; maintenance of 30 mg once daily for up to 6 months.

Eradication of Helicobacter pylori

A. **Amoxicillin, Omeprazole, Clarithromycin (AOC)**
   1. 7-14 days of therapy.
   2. Amoxicillin 1 gm PO qd.
   3. Omeprazole (Prilosec) 20 mg PO bid.
   4. Clarithromycin (Biaxin) 500 mg PO bid.
B. **Metronidazole, Omeprazole, Clarithromycin (MOC)**
   1. 7-14 days of therapy
   2. Metronidazole 500 mg PO bid.
   3. Omeprazole (Prilosec) 20 mg PO bid.
   4. Clarithromycin (Biaxin) 500 mg PO bid.

10. **Symptomatic Medications:**
    -Ondansetron (Zofran) 2-4 mg IV q4h or 8 mg PO q8h prn nausea or vomiting. **OR**
    -Prochlorperazine (Compazine) 5-10 mg IM/IV/PO/PR q4-6h or 25 mg PR q4-6h prn nausea.
11. **Extras:** Upright abdomen, KUB, CXR, ECG, endoscopy. GI consult, surgery consult.
12. **Labs:** CBC, basic metabolic panel, basic chemistry, amylase, lipase. UA, urea breath test for H pylori or stool antigen for H pylori.

Gastrointestinal Bleeding

1. **Admit to:**
2. **Diagnosis:** Upper/lower GI bleed
3. **Condition:**
4. **Vital Signs:** q30min. Call physician if BP >160/90, <90/60; P >120, <50; R>25/min, <10; T >38.5°C; urine output <15 mL/hr for 4h.
5. **Activity:** Bed rest
6. **Nursing:** Place nasogastric tube, then lavage with 2 L of room tempera-

ture normal saline, then connect to low intermittent suction. Repeat lavage q1h. Record volume and character of lavage. Foley to closed drainage; inputs and outputs.

7. **Diet:** NPO
8. **IV Fluids:** Two 16 gauge IV lines. 1-2 L NS over 10-20 minutes; transfuse 2-6 units PRBC as fast as possible.
9. **Special Medications:**
   -Oxygen 2 L by NC.
   -Pantoprazole (Protonix) 80 mg IV over 15min, then 8 mg/hr IV infusion 80 mg IV q12h **OR**
   -Esomeprazole (NexIUM) 20 mg or 40 mg IV or PO once daily.
   -Erythromycin3 mg/kg IV over 20 to 30 minutes, 30 to 90 minutes prior to endoscopy.

Esophageal Variceal Bleeds:
   -Somatostatin (Octreotide) 50 mcg IV bolus, followed by 50 mcg/h IV infusion (1200 mcg in 250 mL of D5W at 11 mL/h).
   -Ceftriaxone (Rocephin) 1 g IV.

10. **Extras:** Portable CXR, upright abdomen, ECG. Surgery and GI consults.
Upper GI Bleeds: Esophagogastroduodenoscopy with band ligation or sclerotherapy; Linton-Nicholas tube for tamponade of esophageal varices.
Lower GI Bleeds: Sigmoidoscopy/colonoscopy (after a GoLytely purge 6-8 L over 4-6h), technetium 99m RBC scan, angiography with embolization.
11. **Labs:** CBC with platelets q4h, troponin, INR. Basic metabolic panel, basic chemistry, ALT, AST, alkaline phosphatase, INR/PTT, type and cross for 4-6 U PRBC and 2-4 U FFP.

Cirrhotic Ascites and Edema

1. **Admit to:**
2. **Diagnosis:** Cirrhotic ascites and edema
3. **Condition:**
4. **Vital Signs:** Vitals q4-6 hours. Call physician if BP >160/90, <90/60; P >120, <50; T >38.5°C; urine output <25 cc/hr for 4h.
5. **Activity:** Bed rest with legs elevated.
6. **Nursing:** Inputs and outputs, daily weights, measure abdominal girth qd, guaiac stool.
7. **Diet:** 2500 calories, 500 mg sodium restriction; fluid restriction to 1-1.5 L/d (if Na <130 mEq/L).
8. **IV Fluids:** Saline lock with flush q shift.
9. **Special Medications:**
   -Spironolactone (Aldactone) 25-50 mg PO qid or 200 mg PO qAM, increase by 100 mg/d to max of 400 mg/d.
   -Diurese to reduce weight by 0.5-1 kg/d (if edema) or 0.25 kg/d (if no edema).
   -Furosemide (Lasix) 40-120 mg PO or IV qd-bid. Add KCL 20-40 mEq PO qAM if renal function is normal **OR**
   -Torsemide (Demadex) 20-40 mg PO/IV qd-bid.
   -Captopril (Capoten) 6.75 mg PO q8h; increase to max 50 mg PO q8h for refractory ascites caused by hyperaldosteronism.
   -Midodrine (Proamatine) 5 mg PO tid and adjust the dose every 24 hours (max 17.5 mg tid) to achieve an increase in systolic BP of 10 to 15 mmHg.
   -Famotidine (Pepcid) 20 mg IV/PO q12h.

-Folic acid 1 mg PO qd.
-Thiamine 100 mg PO qd.
-Multivitamin PO qd.

Paracentesis: Remove up to 5 L of ascites if peripheral edema, tense ascites, or decreased diaphragmatic excursion. If large volume paracentesis, give salt-poor albumin, 6-8 gm for each liter of fluid removed (25 mL of 25% solution); infuse 25 mL before paracentesis and 25 mL 6h after.

10. Symptomatic Medications:
-Docusate (Colace) 100 mg PO qhs.
-Lactulose 30 mL PO bid-qid prn constipation.
-Acetaminophen (Tylenol) 325-650 mg PO q4-6h prn headache.

11. Extras: CXR, abdominal ultrasound, GI consult.

12. Labs: Ammonia, CBC, basic metabolic panel, basic chemistry, LFTs, albumin, amylase, lipase, INR/PTT. Urine creatinine, Na, K. HBsAg, anti-HBs, hepatitis C virus antibody, alpha-1-antitrypsin.

Paracentesis Ascitic Fluid
Tube 1: Protein, albumin, specific gravity, glucose, bilirubin, amylase, lipase, triglyceride, LDH (3-5 mL, red top tube).
Tube 2: Cell count and differential (3-5 mL, purple top tube).
Tube 3: C&S, Gram stain, AFB, fungal (5-20 mL); inject 20 mL into bottle of blood culture at bedside.
Tube 4: Cytology (>20 mL).
Syringe: pH (2 mL).

Acute Hepatitis B

1. Admit to:
2. Diagnosis: Acute hepatitis
3. Condition:
4. Vital Signs: qid. Call physician if BP <90/60; T >38.5°C.
5. Activity:
6. Nursing: Stool isolation.
7. Diet: Clear liquid (if nausea), low fat (if diarrhea).
8. Special Medications:
-Telbivudine (Tyzeka) 600 mg once daily **OR**
-Lamivudine (Epivir HBV) 100 mg/day **OR**
-Adefovir (Hepsera) 10 mg once daily **OR**
-Tenofovir (Viread) 300 mg once daily **OR**
-Entecavir (Baraclude) 0.5-1 mg once daily
-Treat patients with an INR >1.5 or persistent symptoms or bilirubin >10 mg/dL >4weeks.

9. Symptomatic Medications:
-Morphine sulfate 5-10 mg IV/IM q2-4h prn pain.
-Ondansetron (Zofran) 2-4 mg IV q4h or 8 mg PO q8h prn nausea or vomiting.
-Diphenhydramine (Benadryl) 25-50 mg PO/IV q4-6h prn pruritus.

10. Extras: Ultrasound, GI consult.

11. Labs: CBC, basic metabolic panel, basic chemistry, GGT, LDH, amylase, lipase, INR/PTT, IgM anti-HAV, IgM anti-HBc, HBsAg, anti-HCV; alpha-1-antitrypsin, ANA, ferritin, ceruloplasmin, urine copper.

Chronic Hepatitis B

1. Admit to:
2. Diagnosis: Chronic hepatitis B
3. Condition:
4. Vital Signs: qid. Call physician if BP <90/60; T >38.5°C.
5. Activity:
6. Nursing: Stool isolation.
7. Diet: Regular.
8. Special Medications:
   -Entecavir (Baraclude) 0.5 mg to 1 mg once daily **OR**
   -Tenofovir (Viread) 300 mg once daily **OR**
   -Peginterferon alfa-2a, 180 microG once weekly
   -Multivitamin PO qd.
9. Symptomatic Medications:
   -Ondansetron (Zofran) 2-4 mg IV q4h or 8 mg PO q8h prn nausea or
      vomiting. **OR**
   -Diphenhydramine (Benadryl) 25-50 mg PO/IV q4-6h prn pruritus.
10. Extras: Ultrasound, GI consult.
11. Labs: CBC, hepatitis B genotyping, basic chemistry, basic metabolic
   panel, INR/PTT.

Chronic Hepatitis C

1. Admit to:
2. Diagnosis: Hepatitis
3. Condition:
4. Vital Signs: qid. Call physician if BP <90/60; T >38.5°C.
5. Activity:
6. Nursing: Stool isolation.
7. Diet: Clear liquid (if nausea), low fat (if diarrhea).
8. Special Medications:
   -Famotidine (Pepcid) 20 mg IV/PO q12h.
   -Vitamin K 10 mg SQ qd for 3d.
   -Multivitamin PO qd.
9. Symptomatic Medications:
Chronic genotype 1 HCV infection with decompensated cirrhosis:
   -Peginterferon, ribavirin, and sofosbuvir (treatment-naïve patients)
   -Peginterferon alfa-2a,180 micrograms SQ per week. Or peginterferon
      alfa-2b, the dose is 1.5 microgram/kg subcutaneously per week.
      AND
   -Ribavirin (Rebetol) For patients receiving peginterferon alfa-2a, the
      rabinavir dose for patients who weigh 75 kg is 1000 mg/d; or for
      those who weigh >75 kg, 1200 mg/d; divided bid. For patients
      receiving peginterferon alfa-2b, the ribavirin dose for patients weigh-
      ing <65 kg is 800 mg; for 65 to 85 kg 1000 mg; for >85 to 105 kg:
      1200 mg; and for >105 kg: 1400 mg; divided bid. **AND**
   -Sofosbuvir (Solvaldi) 400 mg PO qd.
Treatment-naïve cirrhotic patients with compensated cirrhosis:
   -Sofosbuvir (Solvaldi) 400 mg PO qd. plus peginterferon and ribavirin
      for 12 weeks.

Patients with cirrhosis who have failed prior therapy or cannot use interferon:
-Simeprevir plus sofosbuvir (Solvaldi) 400 mg PO qd.(with ribavirin) for 12 weeks.

Treatment-naïve patients with genotype 2 infection:
-Sofosbuvir (Solvaldi) 400 mg PO qd. and ribavirin for 12 weeks instead of peginterferon and ribavirin for 24 weeks.

For interferon intolerant and non-cirrhotic treatment-experienced patients with genotype 2 infection:
-Sofosbuvir (Solvaldi) and ribavirin for 12 weeks.

Treatment-experienced, cirrhotic genotype 2:
-Sofosbuvir(Solvaldi) 400 mg PO qd. and ribavirin for 12 weeks, sofosbuvir and ribavirin for 16 weeks, or sofosbuvir, peginterferon, and ribavirin for 12 weeks.

Treatment-naïve, interferon intolerant, and non-cirrhotic treatment-experienced with genotype 3 infection:
-Sofosbuvir(Solvaldi) 400 mg PO qd. and ribavirin for 24 weeks.
-Ondansetron (Zofran) 2-4 mg IV q4h or 8 mg PO q8h prn nausea or vomiting.

10. Extras: Ultrasound for hepatocellular carcinoma, GI consult.

11. Labs: CBC, basic metabolic panel, basic chemistry, INR/PTT, HCV genotyping.

Cholecystitis and Cholangitis

1. Admit to:

2. Diagnosis: Bacterial cholangitis

3. Condition:

4. Vital Signs: q4h. Call physician if BP systolic >160, <90; diastolic. >90 mmHg, <60 mmHg; P >120, <50; R>25/min, <10; T >38.5°C.

5. Activity: Bed rest

6. Nursing: Inputs and outputs

7. Diet: NPO

8. IV Fluids: 0.5-1 L LR over 20 min, then D5 ½ NS with 20 mEq KCL/L at 125 cc/h. NG tube at low constant suction. Foley to closed drainage.

9. Special Medications:
-Piperacillin-tazobactam (Zosyn) 3.375 or 4.5 g IV q6h **OR**
-Ticarcillin or piperacillin (Timentin) 3.1 gm IV q4h (single agent) **OR**
-Ceftriaxone (Rocephin) 1 g IV every 24 hours or 2 g IV every 12 hours and metronidazole (Flagyl) 500 mg IV q8h.

10. Symptomatic Medications:
-Morphine sulfate 5-10 mg IV/IM q2-4h prn pain.
-Ketorolac (Toradol) 30-60 mg IM prn pain.
-Ondansetron (Zofran) 2-4 mg IV q4h or 8 mg PO q8h prn nausea or vomiting. **OR**
-Prochlorperazine (Compazine) 5-10 mg IM/IV/PO/PR q4-6h or 25 mg PR q4-6h prn nausea.
-Omeprazole (Prilosec) 20 mg PO bid **OR**
-Famotidine (Pepcid) 20 mg IV/PO q12h.
-Heparin 5000 U SQ q12h **OR**
-Enoxaparin (Lovenox) 30 mg SQ q12h.

11. Extras: CXR, ECG, RUQ ultrasound, HIDA scan, surgical consult.

12. Labs: CBC, basic metabolic panel, basic chemistry, GGT, amylase, lipase, blood C&S x 2. UA, INR/PTT.

Acute Pancreatitis

1. **Admit to:**
2. **Diagnosis:** Acute pancreatitis
3. **Condition:**
4. **Vital Signs:** q1-4h, call physician if BP >160/90, <90/60; P >120, <50; R>25/min, <10; T >38.5°C; urine output < 30 mL/hr for more than 4 hours.
5. **Activity:** Bed rest with bedside commode.
6. **Nursing:** Inputs and outputs, fingerstick glucose qid, guaiac stools. Foley to closed drainage.
7. **Diet:** NPO
8. **IV Fluids:** 1-2 L NS over 1h, then D5 ½ NS with 20 mEq KCL/L at 125 cc/hr.
9. **Special Medications:**
   -Imipenem/meropenem (Primaxin) 0.5-1.0 gm IV q6h for 7 to 10 days if there is necrotizing pancreatitis.
   -Ranitidine (Zantac) 6.25 mg/h (150 mg in 250 mL D5W at 11 mL/h) IV or 50 mg IV q6-8h **OR**
   Famotidine (Pepcid) 20 mg IV q12h.
   -Heparin 5000 U SQ q12h.
   -Total parenteral nutrition should be provided until the amylase and lipase are normal and symptoms have resolved.
10. **Symptomatic Medications:**
    -Morphine sulfate 5-10 mg IV/IM q2-4h prn pain
11. **Extras:** Upright abdomen x-ray, portable CXR, ECG, ultrasound, CT with contrast. Surgery and GI consults.
12. **Labs:** CBC, platelets, basic metabolic panel, basic chemistry, calcium, triglycerides, amylase, lipase, LDH, AST, ALT; blood C&S x 2, hepatitis B surface antigen, INR/PTT, type and hold 4-6 U PRBC and 2-4 U FFP. UA.

Acute Diarrhea

1. **Admit to:**
2. **Diagnosis:** Acute Diarrhea
3. **Condition:**
4. **Vital Signs:** q6h; call physician if BP >160/90, <80/60; P >120; R>25/min; T >38.5°C.
5. **Activity:** Up ad lib
6. **Nursing:** Daily weights, inputs and outputs.
7. **Diet:** Boiled starches and cereals (eg, potatoes, noodles, rice, wheat, and oat) with salt; crackers, bananas, soup, and boiled vegetables. No high fat foods. No lactose-containing foods.
8. **IV Fluids:** 1-2 L NS over 1 hours; then D5 ½ NS with 40 mEq KCL/L at 125 cc/h.

9. Special Medications:
Febrile or gross blood in stool or neutrophils on microscopic exam or prior travel:
-Ciprofloxacin (Cipro) 500 mg PO bid **OR**
-Levofloxacin (Levaquin) 500 mg PO qd **OR**
-Trimethoprim/SMX (Bactrim DS) (160/800 mg) one DS tab PO bid.
Patients with acute diarrhea after use of antibiotics Clostridium difficile:
-Metronidazole (Flagyl) 250 mg PO or IV qid for 10-14 days **OR**
-Vancomycin 125 mg PO qid for 10 days (500 PO qid for 10-14 days).
Listeria monocytogenes:
-Trimethoprim-sulfamethoxazole (one double-strength tablet twice daily) for seven days **OR**
-Ampicillin 1-2 gm IV q4-6h **AND**
Gentamicin or tobramycin 7 mg/kg in 50 mL of D5W over 60 min IV q24h.
Moderate to severe travelers' diarrhea with more than four unformed stools daily, fever, blood, pus, or mucus in the stool.
-Ciprofloxacin 500 mg twice daily OR
-Norfloxacin 400 mg twice daily
-Levofloxacin (Levaquin) 500 mg once daily for three to five days in the absence of suspected EHEC.
-Azithromycin (500 mg PO once daily for three days OR Erythromycin 500 mg PO twice daily for five days.
-Loperamide (Imodium) may be used for patients without fever or bloody stools. Two tablets (4 mg) initially, then 2 mg after each unformed stool.
-Diphenoxylate (Lomotil) 2 tablets (4 mg) four times daily.
-Bismuth subsalicylate (Pepto-Bismol) may be used for patients with significant fever and dysentery. 30 mL or two tablets every 30 minutes for eight doses.
11. Extras: Upright abdomen. GI consult.
12. Labs: SMA7 and 12, CBC with differential, UA, blood culture x 2.
Stool studies: Wright's stain for fecal leukocytes, culture for enteric pathogens, ova and parasites x 3, clostridium difficile toxin, E coli 0157:H7 culture.

Specific Treatment of Acute Diarrhea

Shigella:
-Trimethoprim/SMX, (Bactrim) one DS tab PO bid for 5 days **OR**
-Ciprofloxacin (Cipro) 500 mg PO bid for 5 days **OR**
-Azithromycin (Zithromax) 500 mg PO x 1, then 250 mg PO qd x 4.
Salmonella (bacteremia):
-Ofloxacin (Floxin) 400 mg IV/PO q12h for 14 days **OR**
-Ciprofloxacin (Cipro) 400 mg IV q12h or 750 mg PO q12h for 14 days **OR**
-Trimethoprim/SMX (Bactrim) one DS tab PO bid for 14 days **OR**
-Ceftriaxone (Rocephin) 2 gm IV q12h for 14 days.
Campylobacter jejuni:
-Erythromycin 250 mg PO qid for 5-10 days **OR**
-Azithromycin (Zithromax) 500 mg PO x 1, then 250 mg PO qd x 4 **OR**
-Ciprofloxacin (Cipro) 500 mg PO bid for 5 days.

Enterotoxic/Enteroinvasive E coli (Travelers Diarrhea):
-Ciprofloxacin (Cipro) 500 mg PO bid for 5-7 days **OR**
-Trimethoprim/SMX (Bactrim), one DS tab PO bid for 5-7 days.
Antibiotic-Associated and Pseudomembranous Colitis (Clostridium difficile):
-Metronidazole (Flagyl) 250 mg PO or IV qid for 10-14 days **OR**
-Vancomycin 125 mg PO qid for 10 days (recurrent disease: 500 PO qid for 10-14 days).
Yersinia Enterocolitica (sepsis):
-Trimethoprim/SMX (Bactrim), one DS tab PO bid for 5-7 days **OR**
-Ciprofloxacin (Cipro) 500 mg PO bid for 5-7 days **OR**
-Ofloxacin (Floxin) 400 mg PO bid **OR**
-Ceftriaxone (Rocephin) 1 gm IV q12h.
Entamoeba Histolytica (Amebiasis):
Mild to Moderate Intestinal Disease:
-Metronidazole (Flagyl) 750 mg PO tid for 10 days **OR**
-Tinidazole 2 gm per day PO for 3 days **Followed By:**
-Iodoquinol 650 mg PO tid for 20 days **OR**
-Paromomycin 25-30 mg/kg/d PO tid for 7 days.
Severe Intestinal Disease:
-Metronidazole (Flagyl)750 mg PO tid for 10 days **OR**
-Tinidazole 600 mg PO bid for 5 days **Followed By:**
-Iodoquinol 650 mg PO tid for 20 days **OR**
-Paromomycin 25-30 mg/kg/d PO tid for 7 days.
Giardia Lamblia:
-Quinacrine 100 mg PO tid for 5d **OR**
-Metronidazole 250 mg PO tid for 7 days **OR**
-Nitazoxanide (Alinia) 200 mg PO q12h x 3 days.
Cryptosporidium:
-Paromomycin 500 mg PO qid for 7-10 days [250 mg] **OR**
-Nitazoxanide (Alinia) 200 mg PO q12h x 3 days.

Crohn Disease

1. **Admit to:**
2. **Diagnosis:** Crohn disease.
3. **Condition:**
4. **Vital Signs:** q8h. Call physician if BP >160/90, <90/60; P >120, <50; R>25/min, <10; T >38.5°C
5. **Activity:** Up ad lib.
6. **Nursing:** Inputs and outputs.
7. **Diet:** NPO except for ice chips and medications for 48h, then low residue or elemental diet, no dairy products.
8. **IV Fluids:** 1-2 L NS over 1h, then D5 ½ NS with 40 mEq KCL/L at 125 mL/hr.
9. **Special Medications:**
   -Sulfasalazine (Azulfidine)(2 g/day)
   -Mesalamine (Asacol) 400-800 mg PO tid or mesalamine (Pentasa) 1000 mg (four 250 mg tabs) PO qid.
   -Metronidazole (Flagyl) 250-500 mg PO q6h (10 or 20 mg/kg/day) or the combination of metronidazole and ciprofloxacin 500 mg twice daily for primary or adjunctive therapy of colonic Crohn's disease. .

-Budesonide controlled ileal release (CIR) 9 mg/day for 8 to 16 weeks and then tapered by 3 mg increments over two to four weeks.
-Loperamide (Imodium) 2-4 mg NG/J-tube q6h prn, max 16 mg/d.
-Cholestyramine (Questran) 4 g/day, increase as needed to 12 g/day tid for patients with non-stenosing ileitis who have watery diarrhea.
-Colestipol (Colestid) 2 g 1-2 times/day; maintenance: 2-16 g/day given once or in divided doses; increase by 2 g once or twice daily at 1- to 2-month intervals
-Azathioprine 50 mg/day; may increase to 2.5 mg/kg per day.
-6-mercaptopurine 50 mg/day. If needed, the dose of 6-MP can be increased to a maximum of 2 mg/kg per day.
-Methotrexate 25 mg per week IM. Switched to oral, subcutaneous or intramuscular methotrexate at a dose of 15 mg per week with folic acid 1 mg/day.
-Infliximab (Remicade) 5 mg/kg IV over 2 hours; may repeat at 2 and 6 weeks
-Adalimumab (Humira) 160 mg (4 injections on day 1), then 80 mg 2 weeks later (day 15). Maintenance: 40 mg every other week beginning day 29.
-Certolizumab pegol (Cimzia) induction 400 mg SQ at weeks 0, 2 and 4, then every 4 weeks.

10. **Extras:** CXR, colonoscopy. GI consult.
11. **Labs:** CBC, basic metabolic panel, basic chemistry, Mg, ionized calcium, blood C&S x 2; stool Wright's stain, stool culture for enteric pathogens, C difficile antigen assay, stool ova and parasites x 3.

Ulcerative Colitis

1. **Admit to:**
2. **Diagnosis:** Ulcerative colitis
3. **Condition:**
4. **Vital Signs:** q4-6h. Call physician if BP >160/90, <90/60; P >120, <50; R>25/min, <10; T >38.5°C.
5. **Activity:** Up ad lib in room.
6. **Nursing:** Inputs and outputs. Nasoenteric tube. Intermittent rolling maneuvers every two hours or the knee-elbow position to redistribute gas in the colon.
7. **Diet:** NPO except for ice chips for 24h, then low residue or elemental diet, no dairy products.
8. **IV Fluids:** 1-2 L NS over 1-2h, then D5 ½ NS with 40 mEq KCL/L at 125 cc/hr.
9. **Special Medications:**
   -Mesalamine (Asacol) 400-800 mg PO tid **OR**
   -5-aminosalicylate (Mesalamine) 400-800 mg PO tid or 1 gm PO qid or enema 4 gm/60 mL PR qhs **OR**
   -Sulfasalazine (Azulfidine) 0.5-1 gm PO bid, increase over 10 days as tolerated to 0.5-1.0 gm PO qid **OR**
   -Olsalazine (Dipentum) 500 mg PO bid **OR**
   -Hydrocortisone retention enema, 100 mg in 120 mL saline bid.
   -Methylprednisolone (Solu-Medrol) 10-20 mg IV q6h **OR**
   -Hydrocortisone 100 mg IV q6h **OR**
   -Prednisone 40-60 mg PO qd.
   -Heparin 5000 U SQ q12h.

-Cyclosporine, 2-4 mg/kg/day, IV over 24 hours. Or 2.3-3 mg/kg PO q12h.
-Infliximab (Remicade) 5 mg/kg IV over 2 hours; may repeat at 2 and 6 weeks
-Adalimumab (Humira) 160 mg (4 injections on day 1), then 80 mg 2 weeks later (day 15). Maintenance: 40 mg every other week beginning day 29.
-Certolizumab pegol (Cimzia) induction 400 mg SQ at weeks 0, 2 and 4, then every 4 weeks.
-Prednisolone (30 mg IV every 12 hours) or methylprednisolone (16 to 20 mg IV every eight hours).
10. Symptomatic Medications:
-Acetaminophen (Tylenol) 325-650 mg PO q6h prn fever.
11. Extras: Plain abdominal x-ray, abdominal ultrasound. CXR, colonoscopy, GI consult.
12. Labs: CBC, basic metabolic panel, basic chemistry, Mg, ionized calcium, liver panel, blood C&S x 2; stool Wright's stain, stool for ova and parasites x 3, culture for enteric pathogens. UA.

Parenteral Nutrition

General Considerations: Daily weights, inputs and outputs. Finger stick glucose q6h.
Central Parenteral Nutrition:
-Infuse 40-50 mL/h of amino acid-dextrose solution in the first 24h; increase daily by 40 mL/hr increments until providing 1.3-2 x basal energy requirement and 1.2-1.7 gm protein/kg/d.
Standard solution:

Amino acid solution (Aminosyn) 7-10%	500 mL
Dextrose 40-70%	500 mL
Sodium	35 mEq
Potassium	36 mEq
Chloride	35 mEq
Calcium	4.5 mEq
Phosphate	9 mmol
Magnesium	8.0 mEq
Acetate	82-104 mEq
Multi-trace element formula	1 mL/d
(zinc, copper, manganese, chromium)	
Regular insulin (if indicated)	10-60 U/L
Multivitamin(12)(2 amp)	10 mL/d
Vitamin K (in solution, SQ, IM)	10 mg/week
Vitamin B12	1000 mcg/week
Selenium (after 20 days of continuous TPN)	80 mcg/d

Intralipid 20%, 500 mL/d IVPB; infuse in parallel with standard solution at 1 mL/min for 15 min; if no adverse reactions, increase to 100 mL/hr once daily or 20 mg/hr continuously. Obtain serum triglyceride 6h after end of infusion (maintain <250 mg/dL).
Cyclic Total Parenteral Nutrition:
-12h night schedule; taper continuous infusion in morning by reducing rate to half of original rate for 1 hour. Further reduce rate by half for an additional hour, then discontinue. Finger stick glucose q4-6h; restart TPN in afternoon. Taper at beginning and end of cycle. Final rate of

185 mL/hr for 9-10 h and 2 hours of taper at each end for total of 2000 mL.
7. **Special Medications:**
   -Famotidine (Pepcid) 20 mg IV q12h or 40 mg/day in TPN **OR**
   -Ranitidine (Zantac) 50 mg IV q8h or 150 mg/day in TPN.
8. **Extras:** Nutrition consult.
9. **Labs:**
   Daily labs: SMA7, osmolality, CBC, cholesterol, triglyceride, urine glucose and specific gravity.
   Twice weekly Labs: Calcium, phosphate, SMA-12, magnesium
   Weekly Labs: Serum albumin and protein, pre-albumin, ferritin, INR/PTT, zinc, copper, B12, folate, 24h urine nitrogen and creatinine.

Enteral Nutrition

General Considerations: Daily weights, inputs and outputs, naso-duodenal feeding tube. Head-of-bed at 30° while enteral feeding and 2 hours after completion.

Enteral Bolus Feeding: Give 50-100 mL of enteral solution (Pulmocare, Jevity, Vivonex, Osmolite, Vital HN) q3h. Increase amount in 50 mL steps to max of 250-300 mL q3-4h; 30 kcal of nonprotein calories/kg/d and 1.5 gm protein/kg/d. Before each feeding, measure residual volume, and delay feeding by 1h if >100 mL. Flush tube with 100 cc of water after each bolus.

Continuous enteral infusion: Initial enteral solution (Pulmocare, Jevity, Vivonex, Osmolite) 30 mL/hr. Measure residual volume q1h for 12h then tid; hold feeding for 1h if >100 mL. Increase rate by 25-50 mL/hr at 24 hr intervals as tolerated until final rate of 50-100 mL/hr. Three table-spoonfuls of protein powder (Promix) may be added to each 500 cc of solution. Flush tube with 100 cc water q8h.

Special Medications:
   -Metoclopramide (Reglan) 10-20 mg IV/NG **OR**
   -Erythromycin 125 mg IV or via nasogastric tube q8h.
   -Famotidine (Pepcid) 20 mg IV/PO q12h **OR**
   -Ranitidine (Zantac) 150 mg NG bid.

Symptomatic Medications:
   -Loperamide (Imodium) 2-4 mg NG/J-tube q6h prn, max 16 mg/d **OR**
   -Diphenoxylate/atropine (Lomotil) 1-2 tabs or 5-10 mL (2.5 mg/5 mL) PO/J-tube q4-6h prn, max 12 tabs/d.

Extras: CXR, plain abdominal x-ray for tube placement, nutrition consult.

Labs:
   Daily labs: Basic metabolic profile, basic chemistry, osmolality, CBC, cholesterol, triglyceride.
   Weekly labs: Protein, Mg, INR/PTT, 24h urine nitrogen and creatinine. Pre-albumin, retinol-binding protein.

Hepatic Encephalopathy

1. **Admit to:**
2. **Diagnosis:** Hepatic encephalopathy
3. **Condition:**
4. **Vital Signs:** q1-4h, neurochecks q4h. Call physician if BP >160/90,<90/60; P >120,<50; R>25/min,<10; T >38.5°C.
5. **Allergies:** Avoid sedatives, NSAIDS, amoxicillin-calvulanate, acetaminophen, isoniazid, trimethoprim-sulfamethoxazole, nitrofurantoin valproic acid, niacin.
6. **Activity:** Bed rest.
7. **Nursing:** Keep head-of-bed at 40 degrees; chart stools. Egg crate mattress. Record inputs and outputs. Foley to closed drainage.
8. **Diet:** NPO for 8 hours, then nasogastric enteral feedings at 30 mL/hr. Increase rate by 25-50 mL/hr at 24 hr intervals as tolerated until 50-100 mL/hr.
9. **IV Fluids:** D5W at TKO.
10. **Special Medications:**
    -Lactulose 30-45 mL PO q1h for 3 doses, then 15-45 mL PO bid-qid prnto produce 3 soft stools/d **OR**
    -Lactulose enema 300 mL in 700 mL of tap water; instill 200-250 mL per rectal tube bid-qid **AND**
    -Neomycin 500 mg PO tid or 1 gram twice daily **OR**
    -Rifaximin (Xifaxan) 400 mg taken orally three times daily or 550 mg taken orally two times a day.
    -Ranitidine (Zantac) 50 mg IV q8h or 150 mg PO bid.
    -Multivitamin PO qAM or 1 ampule IV qAM.
    -Folic acid 1 mg PO/IV qd.
    -Thiamine 100 mg PO/IV qd.
11. **Extras:** CXR, ECG; GI and dietetics consults.
12. **Labs:** Ammonia, CBC, platelets, basic metabolic panel, basic chemistry, AST, ALT, GGT, LDH, alkaline phosphatase, protein, albumin, bilirubin, INR/PTT, ABG, blood C&S x 2, hepatitis B surface antibody. UA.

Alcohol Withdrawal

1. **Admit to:**
2. **Diagnosis:** Alcohol withdrawals/delirium tremens.
3. **Condition:**
4. **Vital Signs:** q10 minutes to 1 h. Call physician if BP >160/90, <90/60; P >130, <50; R>25/min, <10; T >38.5°C; or increase in agitation.
5. **Activity:**
6. **Nursing:** Seizure precautions. Soft restraints prn.
7. **Diet:** Regular, push fluids.
8. **IV Fluids:** Saline lock or D5 ½ NS at 100-125 cc/h.
9. **Special Medications:**
Withdrawal syndrome:
    -Chlordiazepoxide (Librium) 50-100 mg slow IV q4-6h until the appropriate level of sedation is achieved. **OR**
    -Diazepam (Valium) IV diazepam , 5 to 10 mg IV every 5 to 10 minutes until the appropriate level of sedation is achieved. **OR**

-Lorazepam (Ativan) 2 to 4 mg IV every 15 to 20 minutes until the appropriate level of sedation is achieved.
-When the withdrawal symptom score is elevated, additional medication is given.

Refractory delirium tremens:
-Phenobarbital can be very effective when given with benzodiazepines 130 to 260 mg IV, repeated every 15 to 20 minutes, until symptoms are controlled.
- Propofol (Diprivan) 2 mg/kg IV push over 2-5 min, then 50 mcg/kg/min; titrate up to 165 mcg/kg/min

Seizures:
-Thiamine 100 mg IV push **AND**
-Dextrose water 50%, 50 mL IV push.
-Lorazepam (Ativan) 0.1 mg/kg IV at 2 mg/min; may repeat x 1 if seizures continue.

Wernicke-Korsakoff Syndrome:
-Thiamine 100 mg IV stat, then 100 mg IV qd.

10. Symptomatic Medications:
-Multivitamin 1 amp IV, then 1 tab PO qd.
-Folate 1 mg PO qd.
-Thiamine 100 mg PO qd.
-Acetaminophen (Tylenol) 1-2 PO q4-6h prn headache.

11. Extras: CXR, ECG. Alcohol rehabilitation and social work consult.

12. Labs: CBC, basic metabolic panel, basic chemistry, Mg, amylase, lipase, liver panel, urine drug screen. UA, INR/PTT.

Toxicology

Poisoning and Drug Overdose

Decontamination:
-**Gastric Lavage:** If less than 2 hours since ingestion, place patient left side down, place nasogastric tube, and check position by injecting 10 mL of water and aspirating. Lavage with normal saline until clear fluid, then leave activated charcoal or other antidote. Gastric lavage is contraindicated for corrosives.
-**Activated Charcoal:** 50 gm PO. Repeat q2-6h for large ingestions.
-**Hemodialysis** for isopropanol, methanol, ethylene glycol, severe salicylate intoxication (>100 mg/dL), lithium, or theophylline.

Antidotes:
  Narcotic Overdose:
  -Naloxone (Narcan) 0.4 mg IV/ET/IM/SC, may repeat q2min.
  Methanol Ingestion:
  -Fomepizole is loaded at 15 mg/kg intravenously, followed by 10 mg/kg every 12 hours, with adjustments for hemodialysis or after more than two days of therapy. Once begun, ADH inhibition with fomepizole should be continued until the diagnosis of toxic alcohol ingestion has been ruled out, or until blood pH is normal and serum alcohol concentration is <20 mg/dL in the presence of retinal or renal injury.
  Ethylene Glycol Ingestion:
  -Fomepizole (Antizol) 15 mg/kg IV, followed by 10 mg/kg q12 hours, with adjustments for hemodialysis or after more than two days of therapy until ethylene glycol level is less than 20 mg/dL **AND**
  -Pyridoxine 100 mg IV q6h for 2 days and thiamine 100 mg IV q6h for 2 days.
  Carbon Monoxide Intoxication:
  -Hyperbaric oxygen therapy or 100% oxygen by mask if hyperbaric oxygen is not available.

Labs: Drug screen (serum, gastric, urine); blood levels, basic metabolic panel, fingerstick glucose, CBC, LFTs, ECG.

Acetaminophen Overdose

1. **Admit to:** Medical intensive care unit.
2. **Diagnosis:** Acetaminophen overdose
3. **Condition:**
4. **Vital Signs:** q1h. Call physician if BP >160/90, <90/60; P >130, <50 <50; R>25/min, <10; urine output <20 cc/h for 3 hours.
5. **Activity:** Bed rest with bedside commode.
6. **Nursing:** Inputs and outputs, aspiration and seizure precautions. Place large bore (Ewald) NG tube, then lavage with 2 L of NS.
7. **Diet:** NPO
8. **IV Fluids:**
9. **Special Medications:**
Gastrointestinal Decontamination: Adult patients who present <4 hours after a potentially toxic ingestion of acetaminophen (single dose ≥7.5 g) should be given activated charcoal, 1 g/kg (max 50 g) by mouth. Char-

coal should be withheld in patients who are sedated, unless endotracheal intubation is performed first. However, endotracheal intubation should not be performed solely for the purpose of giving charcoal.

Acetylcysteine 20 hour IV protocol:
   -Administer acetylcysteine loading dose of 150 mg/kg IV over 15 to 60 minutes (we recommend 60 minutes). Next, administer a 4 hour infusion at 12.5 mg/kg per hour IV. Finally, administer a 16 hour infusion at 6.25 mg/kg per hour IV.

Acetylcysteine 72 hour oral protocol:
   -Give a loading dose of 140 mg/kg PO.
   -Next, give a dose of 70 mg/kg PO every four hours for a total of 17 doses.
   -Ondansetron (Zofran) 2-4 mg IV q4h prn nausea or vomiting.

10. **Extras:** ECG.
11. **Labs:** CBC, basic metabolic panel, basic chemistry, LFTs, INR/PTT, acetaminophen level now and in 4h. UA.

Theophylline Overdose

1. **Admit to:** Medical intensive care unit.
2. **Diagnosis:** Theophylline overdose
3. **Condition:**
4. **Vital Signs:** Neurochecks q8h. Call physician if BP >160/90, <90/60; P >130; <50; R >25/min, <10.
5. **Activity:** Bed rest
6. **Nursing:** ECG monitoring until level <20 mcg/mL, aspiration precautions. Insert single lumen NG tube and lavage with normal saline if recent ingestion.
7. **Diet:** NPO
8. **IV Fluids:** D5 ½ NS at 125 cc/h
9. **Special Medications:**
   -Activated charcoal 50 gm PO q4-6h until theophylline level <20 mcg/mL. Maintain head-of-bed at 30-45 degrees to prevent aspiration of charcoal.
   -Charcoal hemoperfusion if the serum level is >60 mcg/mL or if signs of neurotoxicity, seizure, coma.
   -**Seizure:** Lorazepam (Ativan) 0.1 mg/kg IV at 2 mg/min; may repeat x 1 if seizures continue.
10. **Extras:** ECG.
11. **Labs:** CBC, basic metabolic panel, basic chemistry, theophylline level now and in q6-8h; INR/PTT, liver panel. UA.

Tricyclic Antidepressant Overdose

1. **Admit to:** Medical intensive care unit.
2. **Diagnosis:** TCA Overdose
3. **Condition:**
4. **Vital Signs:** Vial signs q1h.
5. **Activity:** Bedrest.
6. **Nursing:** Continuous suicide observation. ECG monitoring, inputs and outputs, aspiration and seizure precautions. Maintain head-of-bed at 30-45 degree angle to prevent charcoal aspiration. Place single-lumen nasogastric tube and lavage with 2 liters of normal saline if recent ingestion.
7. **Diet:** NPO
8. **IV Fluids:** 1 L NS IV over 30 min, then 100-125 mL/hr.
9. **Special Medications:**
   -Charcoal 1 g/kg of charcoal (up to 50 g) in patients who present within two hours of ingestion unless bowel obstruction, ileus, or perforation is suspected. Charcoal should be withheld in patients who are sedated, unless endotracheal intubation is performed first. Endotracheal intubation, should not be performed solely for the purpose of giving charcoal.
   -Sodium bicarbonate in patients with a QRS interval >100 msec or a ventricular arrhythmia. 1 to 2 mEq/kg given as a rapid IV push through a large bore IV catheter. Two to three vials or prefilled syringes (50 mL each) of 8.4 percent sodium bicarbonate .
   -If the QRS narrows after bolus therapy, infuse 125 to 150 mEq of sodium bicarbonate in 1 liter of D5W at 250 mL/hour in adults.
   -Taper bicarbonate therapy after the resolution of ECG changes by reducing the infusion by about 25 percent per hour over four hours.
   -Arterial blood pH measurements should be obtained during treatment with sodium bicarbonate with a goal pH of 7.50 to 7.55.
   -Magnesium sulfate 1-2 g IV/IO in 10 mL D5W or NS, IV push in unstable patients for wide complex ventricular arrhythmias.
   -Norepinephrine (Levophed) 8-12 mcg/min IV, titrate to systolic 100 mm Hg (8 mg in 500 mL D5W)
11. **Extras:** ECG.
12. **Labs:** Urine toxicology screen, serum TCA level, liver panel, CBC, SMA-7 and 12, UA.

74 Tricyclic Antidepressant Overdose

Neurologic Disorders

Ischemic Stroke

1. **Admit to:**
2. **Diagnosis:** Ischemic stroke
3. **Condition:**
4. **Vital Signs:** Vital signs q1h and neurochecks q1h for 6 hours. Call physician if BP >185/105, <110/60; P >120, <50; R>24, <10; T >38.5°C.
5. **Activity:** Bedrest.
6. **Nursing:** Head-of-bed at 30 degrees, turn q2h when awake, range of motion exercises qid. Foley catheter. Inputs and outputs. Intermittent pneumatic compression device. Bleeding precautions: check puncture sites for bleeding or hematomas.
7. **Diet:** NPO, then dysphagia ground diet with thickened liquids after swallowing study.
8. **IV Fluids:** 0.9% normal saline at 100 cc/h. Oxygen at 2 L per minute by nasal cannula.
9. **Special Medications:**

Ischemic Stroke <4.5 hours:
  a. Tissue plasminogen activator (rt-PA, Alteplase) is indicated if the patient presents within 4.5 hours of onset of symptoms and the stroke is non-hemorrhagic; 0.9 mg/kg, maximum 90 mg. 10% of the dose is given IV over 1 min, and the remainder over 1 h.
  b. Repeat CT scan 24 hours after completion of tPA. Begin heparin if scan results are negative for hemorrhage.
  c. Heparin 12 U/kg/h continuous IV infusion, without a bolus. Check aPTT q6h to maintain 1.2-1.5 x control.

Venous Thromboembolism Prophylaxis:
-Enoxaparin 40 mg daily, starting 24 hours after rtPA **OR**
-Unfractionated heparin 5000 units subcutaneously bid-tid, starting 24 hours after rtPA.

Completed Ischemic Stroke:
-Administer regular insulin 1 unit/hour IV/IO if blood glucose of 140 to 180 mg/dL.
-Aspirin 160-325 mg PO qd. Aspirin should not be given for the first 24 hours following treatment with intravenous or intra-arterial thrombolytic therapy. Intracranial hemorrhage should be excluded by CT scan before starting aspirin. Discharge on aspirin 325 mg PO qd **PLUS** Clopidogrel (Plavix) 75 mg PO qd.
-Atorvastatin (Lipitor) 10 mg PO qhs.
-Sertraline (Zoloft) 50 mg PO QD.

10. **Symptomatic Medications:**
  -Famotidine (Pepcid) 20 mg IV/PO q12h **OR**
  -Esomeprazole (NexIUM) 20 mg or 40 mg IV or PO once daily.
  -Docusate sodium (Colace) 100 mg PO qhs
  -Bisacodyl (Dulcolax) 10-15 mg PO qhs or 10 mg PR prn.
  -Acetaminophen (Tylenol) 650 mg PO/PR q4-6h prn temp >38°C or headache.
11. **Extras:** CXR, ECG, CT without contrast or MRI with gadolinium contrast; echocardiogram, 24-hour Holter monitor; swallowing studies. Physical therapy consult for range of motion exercises; neurology and

rehabilitation medicine consults.
12. **Labs:** CBC, glucose, basic metabolic panel, basic chemistry, fasting lipid profile, VDRL, ESR, INR/PTT, UA. Lupus anticoagulant, anticardiolipin antibody.

Transient Ischemic Attack

1. **Admit to:**
2. **Diagnosis:** Transient ischemic attack
3. **Condition:**
4. **Vital Signs:** q1-4h with neurochecks. Call physician if BP >160/90, <90/60; P >120, <50; R>25/min, <10; T >38.5°C; or change in neurologic status.
5. **Activity:** Up as tolerated.
6. **Nursing:** Guaiac stools.
7. **Diet:** Dysphagia ground with thickened liquids or regular diet.
8. **IV Fluids:** Saline lock with flush q shift.
9. **Special Medications:**
   -Clopidogrel (Plavix) 75 mg PO qd **OR**
   -Aspirin 25 mg/dipyridamole 200 mg (Aggrenox) 1 tab PO bid **OR**
   -Aspirin 325 mg PO qd after the first 48 hours.
   -Dabigatran (Pradaxa) 150 mg twice daily.
10. **Symptomatic Medications:**
    -Famotidine (Pepcid) 20 mg IV/PO q12h.
    -Docusate sodium (Colace) 100 mg PO qhs.
    -Milk of magnesia 30 mL PO qd prn constipation.
    -Acetaminophen (Tylenol) 650 mg PO/PR q4-6h prn temp >38°C or headache.
11. **Extras:** CXR, ECG, CT without contrast; carotid duplex scan, echocardiogram. Neurology consults.
12. **Labs:** CBC, glucose, basic metabolic panel, basic chemistry, fasting lipid profile, VDRL, drug levels, INR/PTT, UA.

Intracerebral Hemorrhage

1. **Admit to:**
2. **Diagnosis:** Intracerebral hemorrhage
3. **Condition:**
4. **Vital Signs:** Vital signs and neurochecks q1-4h. Call physician if BP >185/105, <110/60; P >120, <50; R>24, <10; T >38.5°C; or change in neurologic status.
5. **Activity:** Bedrest.
6. **Nursing:** Head-of-bed at 30 degrees, turn q2h when awake. Foley catheter to closed drainage. Inputs and outputs. Intermittent pneumatic compression device.
   -Keep room dark and quiet; strict bedrest. Neurologic checks q1h for 12 hours.
7. **Diet:** NPO.
8. **IV Fluids and Oxygen:** 0.9% normal saline at 100 mL/h. Oxygen at 2 L per minute by nasal cannula.

9. **Special Medications:**
   -**Fosphenytoin (Cerebyx)** 20 mg/kg IV/IM (at 150 mg/min), then 4-6 mg/kg/day in 2 or 3 doses (150 mg IV/IM q8h). Fosphenytoin is metabolized to phenytoin; fosphenytoin may be given IM.
   -Tranexamic acid (Lysteda) 2000 mg over 20 minutes, followed by 100 mg/hr.
   -Administer regular insulin 1 unit/hour IV/IO if blood glucose of 140 to 180 mg/dL.
   -Propofol (Diprivan) 2 mg/kg IV push over 2-5 min, then 50 mcg/kg/min; titrate up to 165 mcg/kg/min.
   -Mannitol 20 % (1 g/kg) should be given IV over 5 minutes **OR**
   -Hypertonic saline 7.5% is given as a 250-mL IV bolus dose.
   -Acetaminophen (Tylenol) 650 mg PO/PR q4-6h prn temp >38°C or headache.

   Hypertension:
   -Labetalol (Trandate) 10-20 mg IV q15min prn or 1-2 mg/min IV infusion **OR**
   -Nicardipine (Cardene IV) 5 mg/hr IV infusion, increase rate by 2.5 mg/hr every 15 min up to 15 mg/hr (25 mg in D5W 250 mL) **OR**
   -Enalaprilat (Vasotec IV) 1.25- 5.0 mg IV q6h. Do not use in presence of acute myocardial infarction or bilateral renal stenosis.
10. **Extras:** CXR, ECG, CT without contrast; MRI angiogram. Neurology, neurosurgery consults.
11. **Labs:** CBC, basic metabolic panel, basic chemistry, VDRL, UA.

Subarachnoid Hemorrhage

1. **Admit to:**
2. **Diagnosis:** Subarachnoid hemorrhage
3. **Condition:**
4. **Vital Signs:** Vital signs and neurochecks q1-4h. Call physician if BP >185/105, <110/60; P >120, <50; R>24, <10; T >38.5°C; or change in neurologic status.
5. **Activity:** Bedrest.
6. **Nursing:** Head-of-bed at 30 degrees, turn q2h when awake. Foley catheter to closed drainage. Inputs and outputs. Intermittent pneumatic compression device.
   -Keep room dark and quiet; strict bedrest. Neurologic checks q1h for 12 hours.
7. **Diet:** NPO.
8. **IV Fluids and Oxygen:** 0.9% normal saline at 100 mL/h. Oxygen at 2 L per minute by nasal cannula.
9. **Special Medications:**
   -Nimodipine (Nimotop) 60 mg PO or via NG tube q4h for 21d, within 96 hours of stroke.
   -**Fosphenytoin (Cerebyx)** 20 mg/kg IV/IM (at 150 mg/min), then 4-6 mg/kg/day in 2 or 3 doses (150 mg IV/IM q8h). Fosphenytoin is metabolized to phenytoin; fosphenytoin may be given IM.
   -Tranexamic acid (Lysteda) 2000 mg over 20 minutes, followed by 100 mg/hr.
   -Propofol (Diprivan) 2 mg/kg IV push over 2-5 min, then 50 mcg/kg/min; titrate up to 165 mcg/kg/min
   -Administer regular insulin 1 unit/hour IV/IO if blood glucose of 140 to

180 mg/dL.
-Mannitol 20 % (1 g/kg) should be given IV over 5 minutes **OR**
-Hypertonic saline 7.5% is given as a 250-mL IV bolus dose.
-Acetaminophen (Tylenol) 650 mg PO/PR q4-6h prn temp >38°C or headache.

Hypertension:

-Labetalol (Trandate) 10-20 mg IV q15min prn or 1-2 mg/min IV infusion **OR**
-Nicardipine (Cardene IV) 5 mg/hr IV infusion, increase rate by 2.5 mg/hr every 15 min up to 15 mg/hr (25 mg in D5W 250 mL) **OR**
-Enalaprilat (Vasotec IV) 1.25- 5.0 mg IV q6h. Do not use in presence of acute myocardial infarction or bilateral renal stenosis.

10. **Extras:** CXR, ECG, CT without contrast; MRI angiogram. Neurology, neurosurgery consults.
11. **Labs:** CBC, basic metabolic panel, basic chemistry, VDRL, UA.

Seizure and Status Epilepticus

1. **Admit to:**
2. **Diagnosis:** Seizure
3. **Condition:**
4. **Vital Signs:** q6h with neurochecks. Call physician if BP >160/90, <90/60; P >120, <50; R>25/min, <10; T >38.5°C; or any change in neurological status.
5. **Activity:** Bed rest
6. **Nursing:** Finger stick glucose. Seizure precautions with bed rails up; padded tongue blade at bedside. EEG monitoring.
7. **Diet:** NPO for 24h, then regular diet if alert.
8. **IV Fluids:** D5 ½ NS at 100 mL/hr; change to Saline lock when taking PO.
9. **Special Medications:**

Status Epilepticus:

1. Maintain airway.
2. Position the patient laterally. The head and extremities should be cushioned to prevent injury.
3. Give 100% O_2 by mask. Obtain brief history.
4. Secure IV access. Give thiamine 100 mg IV push, then dextrose 50% 50 mL IV push.
5. **Initial Control:**

   Lorazepam (Ativan) 6-8 mg (0.1 mg/kg; not to exceed 2 mg/min) IV at 1-2 mg/min. May repeat 6-8 mg q5-10min (max 80 mg/24h) **OR**
   Diazepam (Valium), 5-10 mg slow IV at 1-2 mg/min. Repeat 5-10 mg q5-10 min prn (max 100 mg/24h).
   Fosphenytoin (Cerebyx) 20 mg/kg IV/IM (at 150 mg/min), then 4-6 mg/kg/day in 2 or 3 doses (150 mg IV/IM q8h). Fosphenytoin is metabolized to phenytoin; fosphenytoin may be given IM.
   If seizures persist, administer phenobarbital 20 mg/kg IV at 50 mg/min, repeat 2 mg/kg q15min up to max of 30-60 mg/kg.
6. **If seizures persist, intubate the patient and give:**
   - Midazolam (Versed) 0.2 mg/kg IV push, then 0.045 mg/kg/hr; titrate up to 0.6 mg/kg/hr **OR**
   -Propofol (Diprivan) 2 mg/kg IV push over 2-5 min, then 50 mcg/kg/min; titrate up to 165 mcg/kg/min **OR**

-Phenobarbital 20 mg/kg IV at 50 mg/min, repeat 2 mg/kg q15min;
  additional phenobarbital may be given, up to max of 30-60 mg/kg.
-Induce coma with pentobarbital 10-15 mg/kg IV over 1-2h, then 1-1.5
  mg/kg/h continuous infusion. Initiate continuous EEG monitoring.

7. Consider Intubation and General Anesthesia

Maintenance Therapy for Epilepsy:

Primary Generalized Seizures – First-Line Therapy:

-Carbamazepine (Tegretol) 200-400 mg PO tid [100, 200 mg]. Monitor
  CBC.
-Phenytoin (Dilantin) loading dose of 400 mg PO, followed by 300 mg
  PO q4h for 2 doses (total of 1 g), then 300 mg PO qd or 100 mg tid or
  200 mg bid [30, 50, 100 mg].
-Divalproex (Depakote) 250-500 mg PO tid-qid with meals [125, 250,
  500 mg].
-Valproic acid (Depakene) 250-500 mg PO tid-qid with meals [250 mg].

Primary Generalized Seizures -- Second Line Therapy:

-Phenobarbital 30-120 mg PO bid [8, 16, 32, 65, 100 mg].
-Primidone (Mysoline) 250-500 mg PO tid [50, 250 mg]; metabolized to
  phenobarbital.
-Felbamate (Felbatol) 1200-2400 mg PO qd in 3-4 divided doses, max
  3600 mg/d [400, 600 mg; 600 mg/5 mL susp]; adjunct therapy;
  aplastic anemia, hepatotoxicity.
-Gabapentin (Neurontin), 300-400 mg PO bid-tid; max 1800 mg/day
  [100, 300, 400 mg]; adjunct therapy.
-Lamotrigine (Lamictal) 50 mg PO qd, then increase to 50-250 mg PO
  bid [25, 100, 150, 200 mg]; adjunct therapy .

Partial Seizure:

-Carbamazepine (Tegretol) 200-400 mg PO tid [100, 200 mg].
-Divalproex (Depakote) 250-500 mg PO tid with meals [125, 250, 500
  mg].
-Valproic acid (Depakene) 250-500 mg PO tid-qid with meals [250 mg].
-Phenytoin (Dilantin) 300 mg PO qd or 200 mg PO bid [30, 50, 100].
-Phenobarbital 30-120 mg PO tid or qid [8, 16, 32, 65, 100 mg].
-Primidone (Mysoline) 250-500 mg PO tid [50, 250 mg]; metabolized to
  phenobarbital.
-Gabapentin (Neurontin), 300-400 mg PO bid-tid; max 1800 mg/day
  [100, 300, 400 mg]; adjunct therapy.
-Lamotrigine (Lamictal) 50 mg PO qd, then increase to 50-250 mg PO
  bid [25, 100, 150, 200 mg]; adjunct therapy.
-Topiramate (Topamax) 25 mg PO bid; titrate to max 200 mg PO bid
  [tab 25, 100, 200 mg]; adjunctive therapy.

Absence Seizure:

-Divalproex (Depakote) 250-500 mg PO tid-qid [125, 250, 500 mg].
-Clonazepam (Klonopin) 0.5-5 mg PO bid-qid [0.5, 1, 2 mg].
-Lamotrigine (Lamictal) 50 mg PO qd, then increase to 50-250 mg PO
  bid [25, 100, 150, 200 mg]; adjunct therapy.

10. Extras: MRI with and without gadolinium or CT with contrast; EEG
  (with photic stimulation, hyperventilation, sleep deprivation, awake and
  asleep tracings); portable CXR, ECG.

11. Labs: CBC, basic metabolic panel, glucose, Mg, calcium, phosphate,
  liver panel, VDRL, anticonvulsant levels. UA, drug screen.

Endocrinologic Disorders

Diabetic Ketoacidosis

1. **Admit to:**
2. **Diagnosis:** Diabetic ketoacidosis
3. **Condition:**
4. **Vital Signs:** q1-4h. Call physician if BP >160/90, <90/60; P >140, <50; R >30, <10; T >38.5°C; or urine output <20 mL/hr for more than 2 hours.
5. **Activity:** Bed rest with bedside commode.
6. **Nursing:** Inputs and outputs. Foley to closed drainage. Record labs on flow sheet.
7. **Diet:** NPO for 12 hours, then clear liquids as tolerated.
8. **IV Fluids:**
   1-2 L NS (≥16 gauge), repeat until hemodynamically stable, then change to 0.45% saline at 125-150 mL/hr; keep urine output >30-60 mL/h.
   Add KCL when serum potassium is <5.0 mEq/L. Concentration: .20-40 mEq KCL/L.
   Use K phosphate, 20-40 mEq/L, in place of KCL if hypophosphatemic.
   Change to 5% dextrose in 0.45% saline with 20-40 mEq KCL/liter when blood glucose is 250-300 mg/dL.
9. **Special Medications:**
   -Oxygen at 2 L/min by NC.
   -Insulin regular (Humulin) 7-10 units (0.1 U/kg) IV bolus, then 7-10 U/h IV infusion (0.1 U/kg/h); 50 U in 250 mL of 0.9% saline; flush IV tubing with 20 mL of insulin solution before starting infusion. Adjust insulin infusion to decrease serum glucose by 100 mg/dL or less per hour. When bicarbonate level is >16 mEq/L and the anion gap is <16 mEq/L, decrease insulin infusion rate by half.
   -When the glucose level reaches 250 mg/dL, 5% dextrose should be added to the replacement fluids with KCL 20-40 mEq/L.
   -Use 10% glucose at 50-100 mL/h if anion gap persists and serum glucose has decreased to less than 100 mg/dL while on insulin infusion.
   -Change to subcutaneous insulin when the anion gap has cleared; discontinue insulin infusion 1-2h after subcutaneous dose.
10. **Symptomatic Medications:**
    -Famotidine (Pepcid) 20 mg IV q12h.
    -Docusate sodium (Colace) 100 mg PO qhs.
    -Acetaminophen (Tylenol) 325-650 mg PO q4-6h prn headache.
11. **Extras:** Portable CXR, ECG.
12. **Labs:** Fingerstick glucose q1-2h. basic metabolic panel q4-6h. SMA 12, pH, bicarbonate, phosphate, amylase, lipase, hemoglobin A1c; CBC. UA, beta-HCG.

Nonketotic Hyperosmolar Syndrome

1. **Admit to:**
2. **Diagnosis:** Nonketotic hyperosmolar syndrome
3. **Condition:**
4. **Vital Signs:** q1h. Call physician if BP >160/90, <90/60; P >140, <50; R>25/min, <10; T >38.5° C.
5. **Activity:** Bed rest with bedside commode.
6. **Nursing:** Input and output measurement. Foley to closed drainage. Record labs on flow sheet.
7. **Diet:** NPO.
8. **IV Fluids:** 2 L NS over 1-2h (≥16 gauge IV catheter), then give 0.45% saline at 125 mL/hr. Maintain urine output ≥50 mL/h.
   -Add 20-40 mEq/L KCL when urine output adequate.
9. **Special Medications:**
   -Insulin regular 2-3 U/h IV infusion (50 U in 250 mL of 0.9% saline).
   -Famotidine (Pepcid) 20 mg IV/PO q12h **OR**
   -Esomeprazole (NexIUM) 20 mg or 40 mg IV or PO once daily.
   -Heparin 5000 U SQ q12h.
10. **Extras:** Portable CXR, ECG.
11. **Labs:** Fingerstick glucose q1-2h x 6h, then q6h. basic metabolic panel, osmolality. SMA 12, phosphate, ketones, hemoglobin A1C, CBC. UA.

Thyroid Storm and Hyperthyroidism

1. **Admit to:**
2. **Diagnosis:** Thyroid Storm
3. **Condition:**
4. **Vital Signs:** q1-4h. Call physician if BP >160/90, <90/60; P >130, <50; R>25/min, <10; T >38.5°C.
5. **Activity:** Bed rest
6. **Nursing:** Cooling blanket prn temp >39°C, inputs and outputs.
7. **Diet:** Regular
8. **IV Fluids:** D5 ½ NS at 125 mL/h.
9. **Special Medications:**

Thyroid Storm and Hyperthyroidism

Subtotal Thyroidectomy: Indicated in patients with large goiter that extends retrosternally, in pregnant patients, and children who have major adverse reaction to medications.
   -Methimazole (Tapazole) 30-60 mg PO, then maintenance of 15 mg PO qd-bid **OR**
   -Propylthiouracil (PTU) 1000 mg PO, then 50-250 mg PO q4-8h, up to 1200 mg/d; usual maintenance dose 50 mg PO tid **AND**
   -Iodide solution (Lugol's solution), 3-6 drops tid; one hour after propylthiouracil **AND**
   -Dexamethasone (Decadron) 2 mg IV q6h **AND**
   -Propranolol 40-160 mg PO q6h or 5-10 mg/h, max 2-5 mg IV q4h or propranolol-LA (Inderal-LA), 80-120 mg PO qd [60, 80, 120, 160 mg].
   -Acetaminophen (Tylenol) 1-2 tabs PO q4-6h prn temp >38°C.
   -Zolpidem (Ambien) 10 mg PO qhs prn insomnia **OR**
   -Lorazepam (Ativan) 1-2 mg IV/IM/PO q4-8h prn anxiety.

10. **Extras:** CXR PA and LAT, ECG, endocrine consult.
11. **Labs:** CBC, basic metabolic panel, basic chemistry; sensitive TSH, free T4. UA.

Myxedema Coma and Hypothyroidism

1. **Admit to:**
2. **Diagnosis:** Myxedema Coma
3. **Condition:**
4. **Vital Signs:** q1h. Call physician if BP systolic >160/90, <90/60; P >130, <50; R>25/min, <10; T >38.5°C.
5. **Activity:** Bed rest
6. **Nursing:** Triple blankets prn temp <36°C, inputs and outputs, aspiration precautions.
7. **Diet:** NPO
8. **IV Fluids:** IV D5 NS TKO.
9. **Special Medications:**

Myxedema Coma and Hypothyroidism:
-Volume replacement with NS 1 L rapid IV over 1 hour, then 125 mL/h.
-Levothyroxine (Synthroid, Levoxine) 300-500 mcg IV, then 100 mcg PO or IV qd.
-Hydrocortisone 100 mg IV loading dose, then 50-100 mg IV q8h.

Hypothyroidism in Medically Stable Patient:
-Levothyroxine (Synthroid, T4) 50-75 mcg PO qd, increase by 25 mcg PO qd at 2-4 week intervals to 75-150 mcg qd until TSH normalized.
11. **Extras:** ECG, endocrine consult.
12. **Labs:** CBC, basic metabolic panel, basic chemistry; sensitive TSH, free T4. UA.

Nephrologic Disorders

Renal Failure

1. **Admit to:**
2. **Diagnosis:** Renal failure
3. **Condition:**
4. **Vital Signs:** q8h. Call physician if QRS complex >0.14 sec; urine output <20 mL/hr; BP >160/90, <90/60; P >120, <50; R>25/min, <10; T >38.5°C.
5. **Allergies:** Avoid magnesium containing antacids, salt substitutes, NSAIDS. Discontinue phosphate, potassium, and magnesium supplements.
6. **Activity:** Bed rest.
7. **Nursing:** Daily weights, inputs and outputs, chart urine output. If no urine output for 4h, in-and-out catheterize. Guaiac stools.
8. **Diet:** Renal diet of high biologic value protein of 0.6-0.8 g/kg, sodium 2 g, potassium 1 mEq/kg, and at least 35 kcal/kg of nonprotein calories.
9. **IV Fluids:** D5W at TKO.
10. **Special Medications:**
    -Consider fluid challenge (to rule out pre-renal azotemia if not fluid overloaded) with 500-1000 mL NS IV over 30 min. In acute renal failure, in-and-out catheterize and check postvoid residual to rule out obstruction.
    -Furosemide (Lasix) 80-320 mg IV bolus over 10-60 min, double the dose if no response after 2 hours to total max 1000 mg/24h, or furosemide 1000 mg in 250 mL D5W at 20-40 mg/hr continuous IV infusion **OR**
    -Torsemide (Demadex) 20-40 mg IV bolus over 5-10 min, double the dose up to max 200 mg/day **OR**
    -Bumetanide (Bumex) 1-2 mg IV bolus over 1-20 min; double the dose if no response in 1-2 h to total max 10 mg/day.
    -Metolazone (Zaroxolyn) 5-10 mg PO (max 20 mg/24h) 30 min before a loop diuretic.
    -Hyperkalemia is treated with sodium polystyrene sulfonate (Kayexalate), 15-30 gm PO/NG/PR q4-6h.
    -Hyperphosphatemia is controlled with calcium acetate (PhosLo), 2-3 tabs with meals.
    -Metabolic acidosis is treated with sodium bicarbonate to maintain the serum pH >7.2 and the bicarbonate level >20 mEq/L. 1-2 amps (50-100 mEq) IV push, followed by infusion of 2-3 amps in 1000 mL of D5W at 150 mL/hr.
    -Adjust all medications to creatinine clearance, and remove potassium phosphate and magnesium from IV. Avoid NSAIDs, nephrotoxic drugs, and excessive fluids.
11. **Extras:** CXR, ECG, renal ultrasound, nephrology and dietetics consults.
12. **Labs:** CBC, platelets, basic metabolic panel, basic chemistry, creatinine, BUN, potassium, magnesium, phosphate, calcium, uric acid, osmolality, INR/PTT.
Urine specific gravity, UA with micro, urine C&S; 1st AM spot urine electrolytes, eosinophils, creatinine, pH, osmolality. 24h urine protein, creatinine, sodium.

Nephrolithiasis

1. **Admit to:**
2. **Diagnosis:** Nephrolithiasis
3. **Condition:**
4. **Vital Signs:** q8h. Call physician if urine output <30 mL/hr; BP >160/90, <90/60; T >38.5°C.
5. **Activity:** Up ad lib.
6. **Nursing:** Strain urine, measure inputs and outputs. Place Foley if no urine for 4 hours.
7. **Diet:** Regular, push oral fluids.
8. **IV Fluids:** IV D5 ½ NS at 100-125 mL/hr (maintain urine output of 80 mL/h).
9. **Special Medications:**
   -Cefazolin (Ancef) 1-2 gm IV q8h
   -Morphine sulfate 5-10 mg IV/IM q2-4h prn pain
   -Hydrocodone/acetaminophen (Vicodin), 1-2 tab q4-6h PO prn pain **OR**
   -Oxycodone/acetaminophen (Percocet) 1 tab q6h prn pain **OR**
   -Acetaminophen with codeine (Tylenol 3) 1-2 tabs PO q3-4h prn pain.
   -Ketorolac (Toradol) 10 mg PO q4-6h prn pain, or 30-60 mg IV/IM then 15-30 mg IV/IM q6h (max 5 days).
   -Zolpidem (Ambien) 10 mg PO qhs prn insomnia.
11. **Extras:** CT scam, CXR, ECG.
12. **Labs:** CBC, SMA 6 and 12, calcium, uric acid, phosphorous, UA with micro, urine C&S, urine pH, INR/PTT. Urine cystine, send stones for X-ray crystallography. 24 hour urine collection for uric acid, calcium, creatinine.

Hypercalcemia

1. **Admit to:**
2. **Diagnosis:** Hypercalcemia
3. **Condition:**
4. **Vital Signs:** q4h. Call physician if BP >160/90, <90/60; P >120, <50; R>25/min, <10; T >38.5°C; or tetany.
5. **Activity:** Encourage ambulation; up in chair at other times.
6. **Nursing:** Seizure precautions, measure inputs and outputs.
7. **Diet:** Restrict dietary calcium to 400 mg/d, push PO fluids.
8. **Special Medications:**
   -1-2 L of 0.9% saline over 1-4 hours until no longer hypotensive, then saline diuresis with 0.9% saline infused at 125 mL/h **AND**
   -Furosemide (Lasix) 20-80 mg IV q4-12h. Maintain urine output of 200 mL/h; monitor serum sodium, potassium, magnesium.
   -Calcitonin (Calcimar) 4-8 IU/kg IM q12h or SQ q6-12h.
   -Etidronate (Didronel) 7.5 mg/kg/day in 250 mL of normal saline IV infusion over 2 hours. May repeat in 3 days.
   -Pamidronate (Aredia) 60 mg in 500 mL of NS infused over 4 hours or 90 mg in 1 liter of NS infused over 24 hours x one dose.
9. **Extras:** CXR, ECG, mammogram.
10. **Labs:** Total and ionized calcium, parathyroid hormone, basic metabolic panel, basic chemistry, phosphate, Mg, alkaline phosphatase,

prostate specific antigen, carcinoembryonic antigen. 24h urine calcium, phosphate.

Hypocalcemia

1. **Admit to:**
2. **Diagnosis:** Hypocalcemia
3. **Condition:**
4. **Vital Signs:** q4h. Call physician if BP >160/90, <90/60; P >120, <50; R>25/min, <10; T >38.5°C.
5. **Activity:** Up ad lib
6. **Nursing:** Inputs and outputs.
7. **Diet:** No added salt diet.
8. **Special Medications:**

Symptomatic Hypocalcemia:
   -Calcium chloride, 10% (270 mg calcium/10 mL vial), give 5-10 mL slowly over 10 min or dilute in 50-100 mL of D5W and infuse over 20 min, repeat q20-30 min if symptomatic, or hourly if asymptomatic. Correct hyperphosphatemia before hypocalcemia **OR**
   -Calcium gluconate, 20 mL of 10% solution IV (2 vials)(90 mg elemental calcium/10 mL vial) infused over 10-15 min, followed by infusion of 60 mL of calcium gluconate in 500 cc of D5W (1 mg/mL) at 0.5-2.0 mg/kg/h.

Chronic Hypocalcemia:
   -Calcium carbonate with vitamin D (Oscal-D) 1-2 tab PO tid **OR**
   -Calcium carbonate (Oscal) 1-2 tab PO tid **OR**
   -Calcium citrate (Citracal) 1 tab PO q8h or Extra strength Tums 1-2 tabs PO with meals.
   -Vitamin D2 (Ergocalciferol) 1 tab PO qd **OR**
   -Calcitriol (Rocaltrol) 0.25 mcg PO qd, titrate up to 0.5-2.0 mcg qid.
   -Docusate sodium (Colace) 1 tab PO bid.
9. **Extras:** CXR, ECG.
10. **Labs:** Basic metabolic panel, basic chemistry, phosphate, Mg. 24h urine calcium, potassium, phosphate, magnesium.

Hyperkalemia

1. **Admit to:**
2. **Diagnosis:** Hyperkalemia
3. **Condition:**
4. **Vital Signs:** q4h. Call physician if QRS complex >0.14 sec or BP >160/90, <90/60; P >120, <50; R>25/min, <10; T >38.5°C.
5. **Activity:** Bed rest; up in chair as tolerated.
6. **Allergies:** Discontinue ACE inhibitors, angiotensin II receptor blockers, beta-blockers, potassium sparing diuretics.
6. **Nursing:** Inputs and outputs. Chart QRS complex width q1h.
7. **Diet:** Regular, no salt substitutes.
8. **IV Fluids:** D5NS at 125 mL/h
9. **Special Medications:**
   -Calcium gluconate (10% solution) 10-30 mL IV over 2-5 min; second dose may be given in 5 min. Contraindicated if digoxin toxicity is sus-

pected. Keep 10 mL vial of calcium gluconate at bedside for emergent use.
- Sodium bicarbonate 1 amp (50 mEq) IV over 5 min (give after calcium in separate IV).
- Regular insulin 10 units IV push with 1 ampule of 50% glucose IV push.
- Kayexalate 30-45 gm PO/NG/PR now and q3-4h prn.
- Furosemide 40-80 mg IV, repeat prn.
- Consider emergent dialysis if cardiac complications or renal failure.

10. Extras: ECG.

11. Labs: CBC, platelets, SMA7, magnesium, calcium, SMA-12. UA, urine specific gravity, urine sodium, pH, 24h urine potassium, urine creatinine.

Hypokalemia

1. **Admit to:**
2. **Diagnosis:** Hypokalemia
3. **Condition:**
4. **Vital Signs:** Vitals, urine output q4h. Call physician if BP >160/90, <90/60; P>120, <50; R>25/min, <10; T >38.5°C.
5. **Activity:** Bed rest; up in chair as tolerated.
6. **Nursing:** Inputs and outputs
7. **Diet:** Regular
8. **Special Medications:**

Acute Therapy:
- KCL 20 mEq in 100 cc saline infused IVPB over 1 hour; or add 40 mEq to 1 liter of IV fluid and infuse over 4 hours.
- KCL elixir 40 mEq PO tid (in addition to IV); max total dose 100-200 mEq/d (3 mEq/kg/d).

Chronic Therapy:
- Micro-K 10 mEq tabs 2-3 tabs PO tid after meals (40-100 mEq/d) **OR**
- K-Dur 20 mEq tabs 1 PO bid-tid.

Hypokalemia with metabolic acidosis:
- Potassium citrate 15-30 mL in juice PO qid after meals (1 mEq/mL).
- Potassium gluconate 15 mL in juice PO qid after meals (20 mEq/15 mL).

9. **Extras:** ECG, dietetics consult.
10. **Labs:** CBC, magnesium, basic metabolic panel, basic chemistry. UA, urine Na, pH, 24h urine for K, urine creatinine.

Hypermagnesemia

1. **Admit to:**
2. **Diagnosis:** Hypermagnesemia
3. **Condition:**
4. **Vital Signs:** q6h. Call physician if QRS >0.14 sec.
5. **Activity:** Up ad lib
6. **Nursing:** Inputs and outputs, daily weights.
7. **Diet:** Regular
8. **Special Medications:**
- Saline diuresis 0.9% saline infused at 100-150 mL/h to replace urine

loss **AND**

-Calcium chloride, 1-3 gm added to saline (10% solution; 1 gm per 10 mL amp) to run at 1 gm/hr **AND**

-Furosemide (Lasix) 20-40 mg IV q4-6h as needed.

-Magnesium of >9.0 mEq/L requires stat hemodialysis because of risk of respiratory failure.

9. Extras: ECG

10. Labs: Magnesium, calcium, basic metabolic panel, basic chemistry, creatinine. 24 hour urine magnesium, urine creatinine.

Hypomagnesemia

1. **Admit to:**
2. **Diagnosis:** Hypomagnesemia
3. **Condition:**
4. **Vital Signs:** q6h
5. **Activity:** Up ad lib
6. **Diet:** Regular
7. **Special Medications:**
   -Magnesium sulfate 4-6 gm in 500 mL D5W IV at 1 gm/hr. Hold if no patellar reflex. (Mg deficit = 0.2 x kg weight x desired increase in Mg concentration; give deficit over 2-3d) **OR**
   -Magnesium sulfate (severe hypomagnesemia <1.0) 1-2 gm (2-4 mL of 50% solution) IV over 15 min, **OR**
   -Magnesium chloride (Slow-Mag) 65-130 mg (1-2 tabs) PO tid-qid (64 mg or 5.3 mEq/tab) **OR**
   -Milk of magnesia 5 mL PO qd-qid.
8. **Extras:** ECG
9. **Labs:** Magnesium, calcium, basic metabolic panel, basic chemistry. Urine Mg, electrolytes, 24h urine magnesium, creatinine.

Hypernatremia

1. **Admit to:**
2. **Diagnosis:** Hypernatremia
3. **Condition:**
4. **Vital Signs:** q2-8h. Call physician if BP >160/90, <70/50; P >140, <50; R>25/min, <10; T >38.5°C.
5. **Activity:** Bed rest; up in chair as tolerated.
6. **Nursing:** Inputs and outputs, daily weights.
7. **Diet:** No added salt. Push oral fluids.
8. **Special Medications:**

Hypernatremia with Hypovolemia:

If volume depleted, give 1-2 L NS IV over 1 hour, then give D5W or ½ normal saline IV to replace half of body water deficit over first 24hours (correct sodium at 1 mEq/L/h), then remaining deficit over next 1-2 days.

Body water deficit (L) = 0.6(weight kg)([Na serum]-140)

Hypernatremia with ECF Volume Excess:
-Furosemide 40-80 mg IV or PO qd-bid.

Hypernatremia with Diabetes Insipidus:
-D5W to correct body water deficit (see above).
-Desmopressin 5 mcg at bedtime, titrated upward in 5 microg increments depending upon the response of the nocturia. The daily maintenance dose is about 5-20 microg qd or bid. Or nasal spray bottle 10 to 20 microg intranasally once or twice a day. Or one-half a 0.1 mg tablet PO at bedtime, increased to 0.1 mg to 0.8 mg in divided doses. Or 1 mcg subcutaneously every 12 hours.

9. **Extras:** CXR, ECG.
10. **Labs**: Basic metabolic panel, basic chemistry, serum osmolality, liver panel, ADH, plasma renin activity. UA, urine specific gravity. Urine osmolality, Na, 24h urine K, creatinine.

Hyponatremia

1. **Admit to:**
2. **Diagnosis:** Hyponatremia
3. **Condition:**
4. **Vital Signs:** q4h. Call physician if BP >160/90, <70/50; P >140, <50; R>25/min, <10; T >38.5°C.
5. **Activity:** Up in chair as tolerated.
6. **Nursing:** Inputs and outputs, daily weights.
7. **Diet:** Regular diet.
8. **Special Medications:**

Hyponatremia with Hypervolemia and Edema (low osmolality <280 mOsm/L, UNa <10 mmol/L: nephrosis, heart failure, cirrhosis):
-Water restrict to 800 mL/d.
-Furosemide 40-80 mg IV or PO qd-bid.

Hyponatremia with Normal Volume Status (low osmolality <280 mOsm/L, UNa <10 mmol: water intoxication; UNa >20: SIADH, diuretic-induced):
-Water restrict to 800 mL/d.
-Conivaptan (Vaprisol) 20 mg in 100 mL of DFW IV over 30 minutes.
-Hypertonic saline 100-500 mL 3% hypertonic saline at 20 mL/hr.
-Salt tablet 9 g PO bid.
-Furosemide 40-80 mg IV or PO qd-bid.
-Tolvaptan (Samsca) 15 mg once daily; after at least 24 hours, may increase to 30 mg once daily to a maximum of 60 mg once daily titrating at 24-hour intervals to a serum sodium concentration of 145 mEq/L.

Hyponatremia with Hypovolemia (low osmolality <280 mOsm/L) UNa <10 mmol/L: vomiting, diarrhea, third space/respiratory/skin loss; UNa >20 mmol/L: diuretics, renal injury, RTA, adrenal insufficiency, partial obstruction, salt wasting:
-If volume depleted, give 1-2 L of 0.9% saline over 1 hour until no longer hypotensive, then 0.9% saline at 125 mL/h or 100-500 mL 3% hypertonic saline at 20 mL/hr.

Severe Symptomatic Hyponatremia:
If volume depleted, give 1-2 L of 0.9% saline (154 mEq/L) over 1 hour until no longer orthostatic.
Determine volume of 3% hypertonic saline (513 mEq/L) to be infused:

Na (mEq) deficit = 0.6 x (wt kg)x(desired [Na] - actual [Na])

$$\frac{\text{Volume of solution (L)}}{\text{Number of hrs}} = \frac{\text{Sodium to be infused (mEq)}}{\text{(mEq/L in solution) x Number of hrs}}$$

-Correct half of sodium deficit intravenously over 24 hours until serum sodium is 120 mEq/L; increase sodium by 12-20 mEq/L over 24 hours (1 mEq/L/h).
-Hypertonic 3% saline 100-300 mL at 20 mL/h, repeated as needed.
9. **Extras:** CXR, ECG, head/chest CT scan.
10. **Labs:** Basic metabolic panel, basic chemistry, osmolality, triglyceride, liver panel. UA, urine specific gravity. Urine osmolality.

Hyperphosphatemia

1. **Admit to:**
2. **Diagnosis:** Hyperphosphatemia
3. **Condition:**
4. **Vital Signs:** qid
5. **Activity:** Up ad lib
6. **Nursing:** Inputs and outputs
7. **Diet:** Low phosphorus diet.
8. **Special Medications:**
Moderate Hyperphosphatemia:
   -Restrict dietary phosphate to 900 mg/d.
   -Sevelamer (Renagel)800-1600 mg 3 times/day with meals
   -Lanthanum (Fosrenol) 1500 mg/day divided and taken with meals; typical increases of 750 mg/day every 2-3 weeks are suggested as needed to reduce the serum phosphate level <6 mg/dL; usual dosage range: 1500-3000 mg.
Severe Hyperphosphatemia:
   -Volume expansion with 0.9% saline 1-2 L over 1-2h.
   -Dialysis.
9. **Extras:** CXR PA and LAT, ECG.
10. **Labs:** Phosphate, basic metabolic panel, basic chemistry, magnesium, calcium. UA, parathyroid hormone.

Hypophosphatemia

1. **Admit to:**
2. **Diagnosis:** Hypophosphatemia
3. **Condition:**
4. **Vital Signs:** qid
5. **Activity:** Up ad lib
6. **Nursing:** Inputs and outputs.
7. **Diet:** Regular diet.
8. **Special Medications:**
Mild to Moderate Hypophosphatemia (1.0-2.2 mg/dL):
   -Sodium or potassium phosphate 0.25 mMoles/kg in 150-250 mL of NS or D5W at 10 mMoles/h.
   -Neutral phosphate (Nutra-Phos), 2 tab PO bid (250 mg elemental phosphorus/tab) **OR**

-Phospho-Soda 5 mL (129 mg phosphorus) PO bid-tid.

Severe Hypophosphatemia (<1.0 mg/dL):

-Na or K phosphate 0.5 mMoles/kg in 250 mL D5W or NS, IV infusion at 10 mMoles/hr **OR**

-Add potassium phosphate to IV solution in place of maintenance KCL; max IV dose 7.5 mg phosphorus/kg/6h.

9. Extras: CXR PA and LAT, ECG.

10. Labs: Phosphate, basic metabolic panel, basic chemistry, Mg, calcium, UA.

Rheumatologic Disorders

Systemic Lupus Erythematosus

1. **Admit to:**
2. **Diagnosis:** Systemic Lupus Erythematosus
3. **Condition:**
4. **Vital Signs:** tid
5. **Allergies:**
6. **Activity:** Up as tolerated with bathroom privileges
7. **Nursing:**
8. **Diet:** No added salt, low psoralen diet.
9. **Special Medications:**
   -Naproxen (Anaprox) 500-1000 mg/day in 2 divided doses; may increase to 1.5 g/day.
   -Celecoxib (CeleBREX)100-200 mg twice daily
   -Hydroxychloroquine (Plaquenil) 400 mg every day or twice daily for several weeks; 200-400 mg/day for prolonged maintenance therapy
   -Prednisone 60-100 mg PO qd. Maintenance 10-20 mg PO qd or 20-40 mg PO qOD **OR**
   -Methylprednisolone (pulse therapy) 500-1000 mg IV over 30 min q12h for 3-5d, then prednisone 50 mg PO qd.
   -Methotrexate 7.5 mg once weekly or 2.5 mg every 12 hours for 3 doses/week
   -Cyclophosphamide 500 mg once every 2 weeks for 6 doses or 500-1000 mg/m 2 once every month for 6 doses
   -Azathioprine 2 mg/kg/day; may reduce to 1.5 mg/kg/day after 1 month (if proteinuria <1 g/day and serum creatinine stable)
   -Mycophenolate 1 g twice daily for 6 months in combination with a glucocorticoid. Maintenance: 0.5-3 g daily.
   -Rtuximab IV infusion: 375 mg/m 2 once weekly for 4 doses
   -Belimumab IV: Initial: 10 mg/kg every 2 weeks for 3 doses; Maintenance: 10 mg/kg every 4 weeks
   -Rituximab IV infusion: 375 mg/m 2 once weekly for 4 doses
   -Cyclosporine Initial: 4 mg/kg/day for 1 month (reduce dose if trough concentrations >200 ng/mL); reduce dose by 0.5 mg/kg every 2 weeks to a maintenance dose of 2.5-3 mg/kg/day
   -Betamethasone dipropionate (Diprolene) 0.05% ointment applied bid.
10. **Extras:** CXR PA, LAT, ECG. Rheumatology consult.
11. **Labs:** CBC, platelets, basic metabolic panel, basic chemistry, INR/PTT, ESR, complement CH-50, C3, C4, C-reactive protein, LE prep, Coombs test, VDRL, rheumatoid factor, ANA, DNA, lupus anticoagulant, anticardiolipin, antinuclear cytoplasmic antibody. UA.

Acute Gout Attack

1. **Admit to:**
2. **Diagnosis:** Acute gout attack
3. **Condition:**
4. **Vital Signs:** tid
5. **Activity:** Bed rest with bedside commode
6. **Nursing:** Keep foot elevated; support sheets over foot; guaiac stools.

7. **Diet:** Low purine diet.
8. **Special Medications:**
    -Naproxen 500 mg twice daily **OR**
    -Indomethacin 50 mg three times daily) **OR**
    -Nabumetone (Relafen) 1000-2000 mg/day; administered once or twice daily; maximum dose: 2000 mg/day **OR**
    -Celecoxib (CeleBREX) 200 mg/day as a single dose or in divided doses twice daily **OR**
    -Prednisone 30 to 50 for one to two days, then taper over seven to ten days. **OR**
    -Methylprednisolone 20 mg twice daily, with stepwise reduction by half of each dose when improvement begins and maintenance of at least 4 mg twice daily for 5 days **OR**
    -ACTH 40 to 80 USP units bid for two days and then once daily.
    -Intraarticular triamcinolone , 40 mg for a large joint (eg, knee), 30 mg for medium joints (wrist, ankle, elbow) and 10 mg for small joints.
    -Colchicine 1.2 mg at the first sign of flare, followed in 1 hour with a single dose of 0.6 mg (max1.8 mg within 1 hour). Maintenance colchicine: 0.5-0.6 mg PO qd-bid.

Hypouricemic Therapy:
    -Colchicine 0.6 mg once or twice daily for patients with normal renal and hepatic function.
    -Allopurinol (Zyloprim) 300 mg PO qd, may increase by 100-300 mg q2weeks up to 800 mg. Initiated after the acute attack **OR**
    -Febuxostat (Uloric) 40 mg once daily. Increase in dose to 80 mg daily if the urate level does not fall to <6 mg/dL after two week **OR**
    -Pegloticase (Krystexxa) 8 mg IV every 2 weeks

9. **Symptomatic Medications:**
    -Famotidine (Pepcid) 20 mg IV/PO q12h.
    -Morphine sulfate 5-10 mg IV/IM q2-4h prn pain **OR**
    -Hydrocodone/acetaminophen (Vicodin), 1-2 tab q4-6h PO prn pain.
    -Docusate sodium (Colace) 100 mg PO qhs.
    -Zolpidem (Ambien) 5-10 mg qhs prn insomnia.
10. **Labs:** CBC, basic metabolic panel, uric acid. UA with micro. Synovial fluid for light and polarizing micrography for crystals; C&S, Gram stain, glucose, protein, cell count. X-ray views of joint.

Commonly Used Formulae

A-a gradient = $[(P_B - PH_2O) FiO_2 - PCO_2/R] - PO_2$ arterial

$= (713 \times FiO_2 - pCO_2/0.8) - pO_2$ arterial

$P_B = 760$ mm Hg; $PH_2O = 47$ mm Hg; $R = 0.8$
normal Aa gradient <10-15 mm Hg (room air)

Arterial oxygen capacity = (Hgb(gm)/100 mL) x 1.36 mL O_2/gm Hgb

Arterial O_2 content = 1.36(Hgb)(SaO_2)+0.003(PaO_2)= NL 20 vol%

O_2 delivery = CO x arterial O_2 content = NL 640-1000 mL O_2/min

Cardiac output = HR x stroke volume

CO L/min = $\dfrac{125 \text{ mL } O_2/\text{min}/M^2}{8.5\{(1.36)(Hgb)(SaO_2) - (1.36)(Hgb)(SvO_2)\}} \times 100$

Normal CO = 4-6 L/min

Na (mEq) deficit = 0.6 x (wt kg) x (desired [Na] - actual [Na])

SVR = $\dfrac{MAP - CVP}{CO_{L/min}}$ x 80 = NL 800-1200 dyne/sec/cm^2

PVR = $\dfrac{PA - PCWP}{CO_{L/min}}$ x 80 = NL 45-120 dyne/sec/cm^2

GFR mL/min = $\dfrac{(140 - age) \times \text{ideal weight in kg}}{\substack{72 \text{ (males) x serum creatinine (mg/dL)}\\85 \text{ (females) x serum creatinine (mg/dL)}}}$

Creatinine clearance = $\dfrac{U \text{ creatinine (mg/100 mL) x U vol (mL)}}{P \text{ creatinine (mg/100 mL) x time (1440 min for 24h)}}$

Normal creatinine clearance = 100-125 mL/min(males), 85-105(females)

Body water deficit (L) = $\dfrac{0.6(\text{weight kg})([\text{measured serum Na}]-140)}{140}$

Serum Osmolality = 2 [Na] + $\dfrac{BUN}{2.8}$ + $\dfrac{Glucose}{18}$ = 270-290 mOsm/L

Na (mEq) deficit = 0.6 x (wt kg)x(desired [Na] - actual [Na])

Fractional excreted Na = $\dfrac{U \text{ Na/ Serum Na x 100}}{U \text{ creatinine/ Serum creatinine}}$ = NL<1%

Anion Gap = Na - (Cl + HCO_3)

For each 100 mg/dL increase in glucose, Na decreases by 1.6 mEq/L.

Corrected serum Ca$^+$ (mg/dL) = measured Ca mg/dL + 0.8 x (4 - albumin g/dL)

Predicted Maximal Heart Rate = 220 - age

Normal ECG Intervals (sec)

PR	0.12-0.20
QRS	0.06-0.08
Heart rate/min	**Q-T**
60	0.33-0.43
70	0.31-0.41
80	0.29-0.38
90	0.28-0.36
100	0.27-0.35

Total Parenteral Nutrition Equations:

Caloric Requirements: (Harris-Benedict Equations)
Basal energy expenditure (BEE)
  Females: 655 + (9.6 x wt in kg) + (1.85 x ht in cm) - (4.7 x age)
  Males: 66 + (13.7 x wt in kg) + (5 x ht in cm) - (6.8 x age)

A. BEE x 1.2 = Caloric requirement for minimally stressed patient
B. BEE x 1.3 = Caloric requirement for moderately stressed patient (inflammatory bowel disease, cancer, surgery)
C. BEE x 1.5 = Caloric requirement for severely stressed patient (major sepsis, burns, AIDS, liver disease)
D. BEE x 1.7 = Caloric requirement for extremely stressed patient (traumatic burns >50%, open head trauma, multiple stress)

Protein Requirements:
A. Protein requirement for non-stressed patient = 0.8 gm protein/kg.
B. Protein requirement for patients with decreased visceral protein states (hypoalbuminemia), recent weight loss, or hypercatabolic states = 1.0-1.5 gm protein/kg.

Estimation of Ideal Body Weight:
A. Females: 5 feet (allow 100 lbs) + 5 lbs for each inch over 5 feet
B. Males: 5 feet (allow 106 lbs) + 6 lbs for each inch over 5 feet

Commonly Used Drug Levels

Drug	Therapeutic Range
Amikacin	Peak 25-30; trough <10 mcg/mL
Amiodarone	1.0-3.0 mcg/mL
Amitriptyline	100-250 ng/mL
Carbamazepine	4-10 mcg/mL
Desipramine	150-300 ng/mL
Digoxin	0.8-2.0 ng/mL
Disopyramide	2-5 mcg/mL
Doxepin	75-200 ng/mL
Flecainide	0.2-1.0 mcg/mL
Gentamicin	Peak 6.0-8.0; trough <2.0 mcg/mL
Imipramine	150-300 ng/mL
Lidocaine	2-5 mcg/mL
Lithium	0.5-1.4 mEq/L
Mexiletine	1.0-2.0 mcg/mL
Nortriptyline	50-150 ng/mL
Phenobarbital	10-30 mEq/mL
Phenytoin	8-20 mcg/mL
Procainamide	4.0-8.0 mcg/mL
Quinidine	2.5-5.0 mcg/mL
Salicylate	15-25 mg/dL
Streptomycin	Peak 10-20; trough <5 mcg/mL
Theophylline	8-20 mcg/mL
Tocainide	4-10 mcg/mL
Valproic acid	50-100 mcg/mL
Vancomycin	Peak 30-40; trough <10 mcg/mL

Extended Interval Gentamicin and Tobramycin Dosing

Estimate the glomerular filtration rate as follows:

Estimated GFR (mL/min) for males =
$$\frac{(140 - \text{age}) \times \text{ideal weight in kg}}{72 \times \text{serum creatinine (mg/dL)}}$$

Estimated GFR (mL/min) for females =
$$\frac{(140 - \text{age}) \times \text{ideal weight in kg}}{85 \times \text{serum creatinine (mg/dL)}}$$

Extended Interval Gentamicin/Tobramycin Therapy	
GFR (mL/min)	Gentamicin/Tobramycin Dosage Frequency
>60	7 mg/kg every 24 hours
40-59	7 mg/kg every 36 hours
20-39	7 mg/kg every 48 hours
<20	Extended interval not recommended

Each dose is administer over 60 minutes. Therapeutic range is a peak level of 20-30 mcg/mL and a trough level of <1.0 mcg/mL (during the 4 hours before the next dose). Monitor renal function and hearing status.

QT Interval Prolonging Drugs

Amiodarone
Bepridil
Chlorpromazine
Desipramine
Disopyramide
Dofetilide
Droperidol
Erythromycin
Flecainide
Fluoxetine
Foscarnet
Fosphenytoin

Gatifolixin
Halofantrine
Haloperidol
Ibutilide
Isradipine
Mesoridazine
Moxifloxacin
Naratriptan
Nicardipine
Octreotide
Pentamidine
Pimozide
Probucol
Procainamide

Quetiapine
Quinidine
Risperidone
salmeterol
Sotalol
Sparfloxacin
Sumatriptan
Tamoxifen
Thioridazine
Venlafaxine
Zolmitriptan

Commonly Used Abbreviations

⁺/2 NS	0.45% saline solution		hemoglobin, hematocrit, red blood cell indices, white blood cell count, and platelets
ac	ante cibum (before meals)		
ABG	arterial blood gas	cc	cubic centimeter
ac	before meals	CCU	coronary care unit
ACTH	adrenocorticotropic hormone	cm	centimeter
ad lib	ad libitum (desired)	CMF	cyclophosphamide, methotrexate, fluorouracil
ADH	antidiuretic hormone	CNS	central nervous system
		CO₂	carbon dioxide
AFB	acid-fast bacillus	COPD	chronic obstructive pulmonary disease
alk phos	alkaline phosphatase	CPK-MB	myocardial-specific CPK isoenzyme
ALT	alanine aminotransferase	CPR	cardiopulmonary resuscitation
am	morning	CSF	cerebrospinal fluid
AMA advice	against medical	CT	computerized tomography
amp	ampule	CVP	central venous pressure
AMV	assisted mandatory ventilation; assist mode ventilation	CXR	Chest X-ray
		d/c	discharge; discontinue
ANA	antinuclear antibody	D5W	5% dextrose water solution; also D10W, D50W
ante	before		
AP	anteroposterior	DIC	disseminated intravascular coagulation
ARDS	adult respiratory distress syndrome		
ASA	acetylsalicylic acid	diff	differential count
AST	aspartate aminotransferase	DKA	diabetic ketoacidosis
		dL	deciliter
bid	bis in die (twice a day)	DOSS	docusate sodium sulfosuccinate
B-12	vitamin B-12 (cyanocobalamin)	DTs	delirium tremens
		ECG	electrocardiogram
BM	bowel movement	ER	emergency room
BP	blood pressure	ERCP	endoscopic retrograde cholangiopancreatography
BUN	blood urea nitrogen		
c/o	complaint of	ESR	erythrocyte sedimentation rate
c̄	cum (with)		
C and S	culture and sensitivity	ET	endotracheal tube
		ETOH	alcohol
C	centigrade	FEV₁	forced expiratory volume (in one second)
Ca	calcium		
cap	capsule	FiO₂	fractional inspired oxygen
CBC	complete blood count; includes	g gram(s)	

100 Commonly Used Abbreviations

GC	gonococcal; gonococcus		bowels)
GFR	glomerular filtration rate	L	liter
		LDH	lactate dehydrogenase
GI	gastrointestinal	LDL	low-density lipoprotein
gm	gram	liq	liquid
gt	drop	LLQ	left lower quadrant
gtt	drops	LP	lumbar puncture, low potency
h	hour		
H₂0	water	LR	lactated Ringer's (solution)
HBsAG	hepatitis B surface antigen		
HCO₃	bicarbonate	MB	myocardial band
Hct	hematocrit	MBC	minimal bacterial concentration
HDL	high-density lipoprotein		
Hg	mercury	mcg	microgram
Hgb	hemoglobin concentration	mEq	milliequivalent
		mg	milligram
HIV	human immunodeficiency virus	Mg	magnesium
		MgSO₄	Magnesium Sulfate
hr	hour	MI	myocardial infarction
hs	hora somni (bedtime, hour of sleep)	MIC	minimum inhibitory concentration
		mL	milliliter
		mm	millimeter
IM	intramuscular	MOM	Milk of Magnesia
I and O	intake and output-measurement of the patient's intake and output	MRI	magnetic resonance imaging
		Na	sodium
		NaHCO₃	sodium bicarbonate
		Neuro	neurologic
		NG	nasogastric
IU	international units	NKA	no known allergies
ICU	intensive care unit	NPH	neutral protamine Hagedorn (insulin)
IgM	immunoglobulin M		
IMV	intermittent mandatory ventilation	NPO	nulla per os (nothing by mouth)
INH	isoniazid	NS	normal saline solution (0.9%)
INR	International normalized ratio		
		NSAID	nonsteroidal anti-inflammatory drug
IPPB	intermittent positive-pressure breathing		
		O₂	oxygen
		OD	right eye
IV	intravenous or intravenously	oint	ointment
		OS	left eye
IVP	intravenous pyelogram; intravenous piggyback	Osm	osmolality
		OT	occupational therapy
		OTC	over the counter
K⁺	potassium	OU	each eye
kcal	kilocalorie	oz	ounce
KCL	potassium chloride	p, post	after
		pc	post cibum (after meals)
KPO₄	potassium phosphate		
		PA	posteroanterior; pulmonary artery
KUB	X-ray of abdomen (kidneys, ureters,		
		PaO₂	arterial oxygen pres-

	sure		atrial
pAO_2	partial pressure of oxygen in alveolar gas	Resp	respiratory rate
		RL	Ringer's lactated solution (also LR)
PB	phenobarbital	ROM	range of motion
pc	after meals	rt	right
pCO_2	partial pressure of carbon dioxide	s	sine (without)
		s/p	status post
PEEP	positive end-expiratory pressure	sat	saturated
		SBP	systolic blood pressure
per	by	SC	subcutaneously
pH	hydrogen ion concentration (H+)	SIADH	syndrome of inappropriate antidiuretic hormone
PID	pelvic inflammatory disease		
		SL	sublingually under tongue
pm	afternoon		
PO	orally, per os	SLE	systemic lupus erythematosus
pO_2	partial pressure of oxygen		
polys	polymorphonuclear leukocytes	SMA-12	sequential multiple analysis; a panel of 12 chemistry tests. Tests include Na^+, K^+, HCO3, chloride, BUN, glucose, creatinine, bilirubin, calcium, total protein, albumin, alkaline phosphatase.
PPD	purified protein derivative		
PR	per rectum		
prn	pro re nata (as needed)		
PT	physical therapy; prothrombin time		
		SMX	sulfamethoxazole
PTCA	percutaneous transluminal coronary angioplasty	sob	shortness of breath
		sol	solution
		SQ	under the skin
PTT	partial thromboplastin time	ss	one-half
		STAT	statim (immediately)
		susp	suspension
PVC	premature ventricular contraction	tid	ter in die (three times a day)
q	quaque (every)	T4	Thyroxine level (T4)
	q6h, q2h every 6 hours; every 2 hours	tab	tablet
		TB	tuberculosis
		Tbsp	tablespoon
qid	quarter in die (four times a day)	Temp	temperature
		TIA	transient ischemic attack
qAM	every morning		
qd	quaque die (every day)	tid	three times a day
		TKO	to keep open, an infusion rate (500 mL/24h)
qh	every hour		
qhs	every night before bedtime	TMP-SMX	trimethoprim-sulfamethoxazole combination
qid	4 times a day		
qOD	every other day	TPA	tissue plasminogen activator
qs	quantity sufficient		
R/O	rule out	TSH	thyroid-stimulating hormone
RA	rheumatoid arthritis; room air; right		
		tsp	teaspoon

U	units
UA	urinalysis
URI	upper respiratory infection
Ut Dict	as directed
UTI	urinary tract infection
VAC	vincristine, adriamycin, and cyclophosphamide
vag	vaginal
VC	vital capacity
VDRL	Venereal Disease Research Laboratory
VF	ventricular function
V fib	ventricular fibrillation
VLDL	very low-density lipoprotein
Vol	volume
VS	vital signs
VT	ventricular tachycardia
W	water
WBC	white blood count
x	times

Index